MENIERE MAN
IN THE KITCHEN

SUPER
COOKING

New Revised and Updated
Second Edition of
Meniere Man In The Kitchen Book 2

PAGE ADDIE PRESS
UNITED KINGDOM. AUSTRALIA.

Meniere Man In The Kitchen. Super Cooking. ISBN 978-0-6453222-3-1
(Revised and Updated Second Edition of Meniere Man In The Kitchen Book 2)
Published by Page Addie Great Britain, Australia.

BIC Subject category: VFJB A catalogue record for this book is available from the British Library. 1. meniere's disease. 2. meniere. 3. vertigo. 4. dizziness. 5. low sodium. 6. inner ear.

CONTENTS

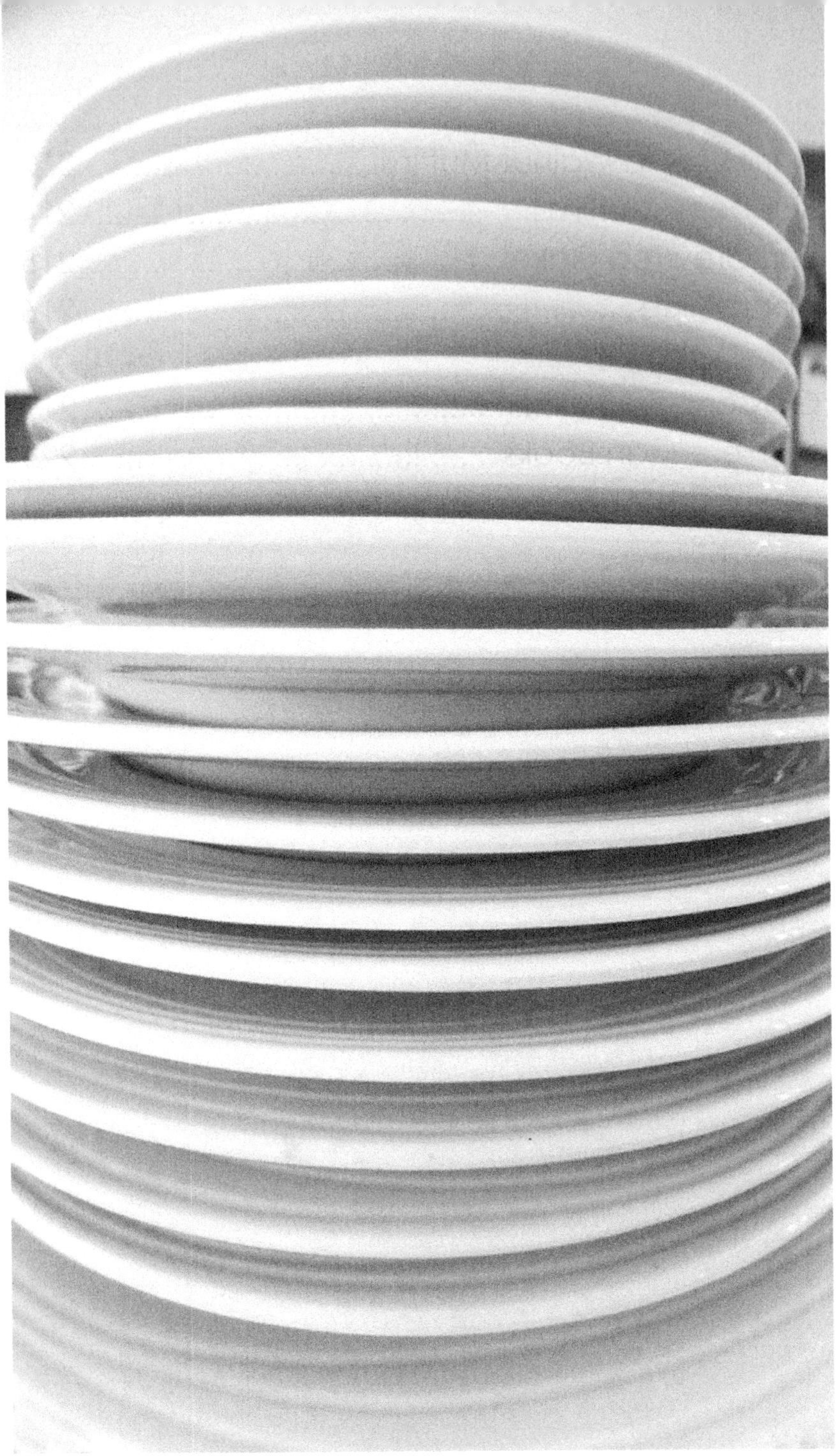

ALL IN THE FAMILY

'Meniere Man in the Kitchen' series is for people who love good food and love cooking. I have a strong conviction that good food and good heath are compatible. Before I was diagnosed with Meniere's, I was a heavy salt user. If my taste buds could have said two words, you would have heard them shout "More salt!" Salt is hard to give up because it's a vehicle for flavor. Low salt diets often fail because just taking salt out of dishes makes the food tasteless. Boring food puts your taste buds to sleep. Eating should be a pleasure not taken as a spoonful of medicine. That's why Meniere Man in the Kitchen is all about recipes that are not only low in salt, but really delicious in flavor.

Cutting down on salt does not have to be an exact science. In the 'Meniere Man in the Kitchen' series, we don't add salt. We don't use foods high in salt or containing hidden salt. We don't count salt grams. There is a good reason for this. From personal experience, focusing on every salt gram over months became a stressful exercise—and current research now shows, that the stress of counting salt grams is something to avoid as much as the salt shaker. Recent research shows, that anxiety from counting salt grams, increases the body's craving for salty foods. In fact, stress actually makes your body retain salt. Dr. Gregory Harshfield of Georgia Health Sciences University says, "Every time a person is stressed, they hold onto as much salt as you get when you eat a small order of French fries. And this can occur many times over the course of a day".

When I had to eat a low salt diet, I also became aware of the frustrations of preparing tasty meals without salt. The question was can 'lack' of salt coexist with delicious flavors? Yes it could. By adapting and testing new versions of family recipes, I went on to change the salt habit of a lifetime. I believe that the change in my diet, was one of the major factors in getting over Meniere's disease. Now, eating tasty, gutsy food without salt, is truly one of life's great pleasures.

Recipes are like friends. You can never have enough of them! I hope you enjoy this revised and updated edition of Book 2, now titled *'Super Cooking'* and enjoy the recipes as much as we do.

TEN LOW SALT COOKING TIPS

Cooking is a creative process and ingredients are interchangeable. If you don't have a specific ingredient, use the glossary in this book to find a substitute. When you do this, you'll create a signature dish of your own.

You can use the recipes in this book to whip up a meal with a minimum of fuss. By using fresh foods, preferably organic, you can cook dishes that taste great without salt. So, as much as possible, eat what is in season. Grow your own herbs. Use shelf fresh spices. Shop in local markets for seasonal produce.

1. Use herbs and spices instead of salt.

2. Marinades and sauces don't have to include salt, soy sauce, barbecue sauce, or fish sauce. Leave them out.

3. Let stocks, soups and stews cook slowly or on

simmer to enhance flavor.

4. Cook stews and casseroles the day before and reheat the next day to increase flavor intensity.
5. Use stocks or wine instead of water in casseroles, soups and braised dishes.
6. Cook grains like rice and beans in stock; add herbs, garlic, and onions for a rich flavor.
7. De-fat pan juices which are left after cooking. Then simply add wine or water to de-glaze the frying pan on low heat. Use these juices as a flavorful sauce.
8. Make sauces from reduced meat or vegetable stocks. Add fresh herbs, season with pepper and thicken with corn flour.
9. Cook with condiments like homemade no salt added chutneys and preserves to give a glaze to roasted meats, grilled or barbecued food.
10. Don't throw out your favorite old recipes. Use the sections in this book to substitute other ingredients for salt and enjoy your familiar flavors.

THE HEALTHY PANTRY

30 LOW SALT ITEMS TO STOCK YOUR FRIDGE, FREEZER OR PANTRY

1. Homemade no salt chicken stock, meat and vegetable stock
2. Dairy: yogurt, butter, eggs
3. No salt homemade mozzarella, ricotta cheese, mascarpone, crème fraiche
4. Fresh herbs. (Grow in containers or in the garden)
5. Rice, pasta of all shapes
6. Beans, lentils and dried legumes, grains
7. Oil for cooking: olive oil
8. Oil for flavor: cold-pressed walnut, extra virgin olive oil, hazelnut, sesame
9. Tomato paste, tomato puree, tinned tomatoes
10. Vinegars: red, white, balsamic, herb infused
11. Onions, shallots, green onions, garlic, ginger

12. Lemons, limes, oranges
13. Long-life vegetables: pumpkin, potatoes
14. Whole grain bread
15. Organic unbleached white flour
16. Low sodium baking powder
17. Nuts: hazelnuts, almonds.
18. Rolled oats
19. Black, white, green and dried peppercorns
20. Mushrooms: Porcini, button, brown, Portobello
21. Homemade no salt tomato sauce, barbecue sauce, chutneys
22. Wines: red and white
23. Salt free corn chips and crackers
24. Grains, wheat, couscous
25. Frozen berries: strawberries, blueberries, raspberries, and blackberries
26. Frozen organic chicken, organic steak, wild caught salmon fillets, wild caught white fish
27. Seasonal vegetables to keep in the fridge: carrots, lettuces, rocket leaves, baby spinach, celery and beetroot
28. In the freezer: no salt pizza bases
29. Exotic ingredients: quince paste, vanilla bean
30. Frozen vegetables: peas, sugar peas, soya beans, green beans

THE HOME DAIRY

No Salt Mozzarella Cheese

One slice of bought whole milk mozzarella can contain 178mg of sodium. One slice of bought low sodium mozzarella contains 5mg. Here is a recipe for homemade no salt mozzarella. You can make this recipe in 30 minutes. Less than the time it takes to go to the supermarket.

Makes: about 500g
Cooking time: 30 minutes

Ingredients

4.5 liters of whole milk

1 1/2 tsp citric acid

1/4 tablet rennet

mineral water

* Do not use junket rennet for making mozzarella, as it is not strong enough.

Method

Mix citric acid in 1 cup cold water.

Pour milk into a heavy bottomed saucepan. Stir in citric acid mixture.

Heat the milk to 32 degrees C, stirring constantly. Remove from heat. Dissolve rennet tablet in 1/4 cup cool water. Add this slowly to the milk using an up and down motion with a slotted metal spoon. Cover with a lid. Let stand for 5 minutes. Remove lid and check the curd. It should resemble custard when pressed lightly with your finger.

Take a metal knife or spatula. Slice across the surface of the curd cutting the curd into 3cm squares. Return the saucepan to the heat and heat the curd to 40 degrees C, while slowly stirring the curd with your spoon. Remove from heat and stir for 2-5 minutes. The more you stir the firmer the mozzarella will be. Pour into a sieve or colander. The curds will drain off from the whey (the liquid). Pour curds into a microwavable bowl. Tip bowl to drain off whey. Microwave on high for 1 minute. Drain off the whey again. Microwave again for 30 seconds. Remove from bowl and place curds on a workbench. Knead, as you would bread dough, turning the cheese and folding the cheese over. Keep kneading until the cheese turns glossy. If cheese doesn't hold together, microwave for another 30 seconds on high.

Cheese is ready when it is so elastic that you can stretch it into a long strand.

Form the cheese into a loaf shape or a ball. You can plait the cheese also. Then fill a bowl with cool water and submerge the cheese for 15 minutes. This will help the cheese keep its shape and maintain a silky texture.

Cheese keeps in the fridge in a covered container for up to 2 weeks. You can also wrap the cheese tightly in cling film and freeze it.

Hot Water Bath Directions

If you don't have a microwave you can create mozzarella by using the following method. Follow cheese-making steps in the recipe up to the microwave instructions. Instead of using the microwave, heat water in a heavy saucepan to 82 degrees C. Spoon the curds into a colander or sieve, folding the curds over gently as you drain off the whey. Dip the colander into the hot water several times. Take a spoon and fold the curds until they become elastic and pliable. Remove the curds, stretch and pull. If it does not stretch easily, return to the hot water bath in the colander and repeat the process. Then continue kneading cheese until it is pliable like long elastic. Submerge in water for 15 minutes. Drain. Store covered in the fridge as directed.

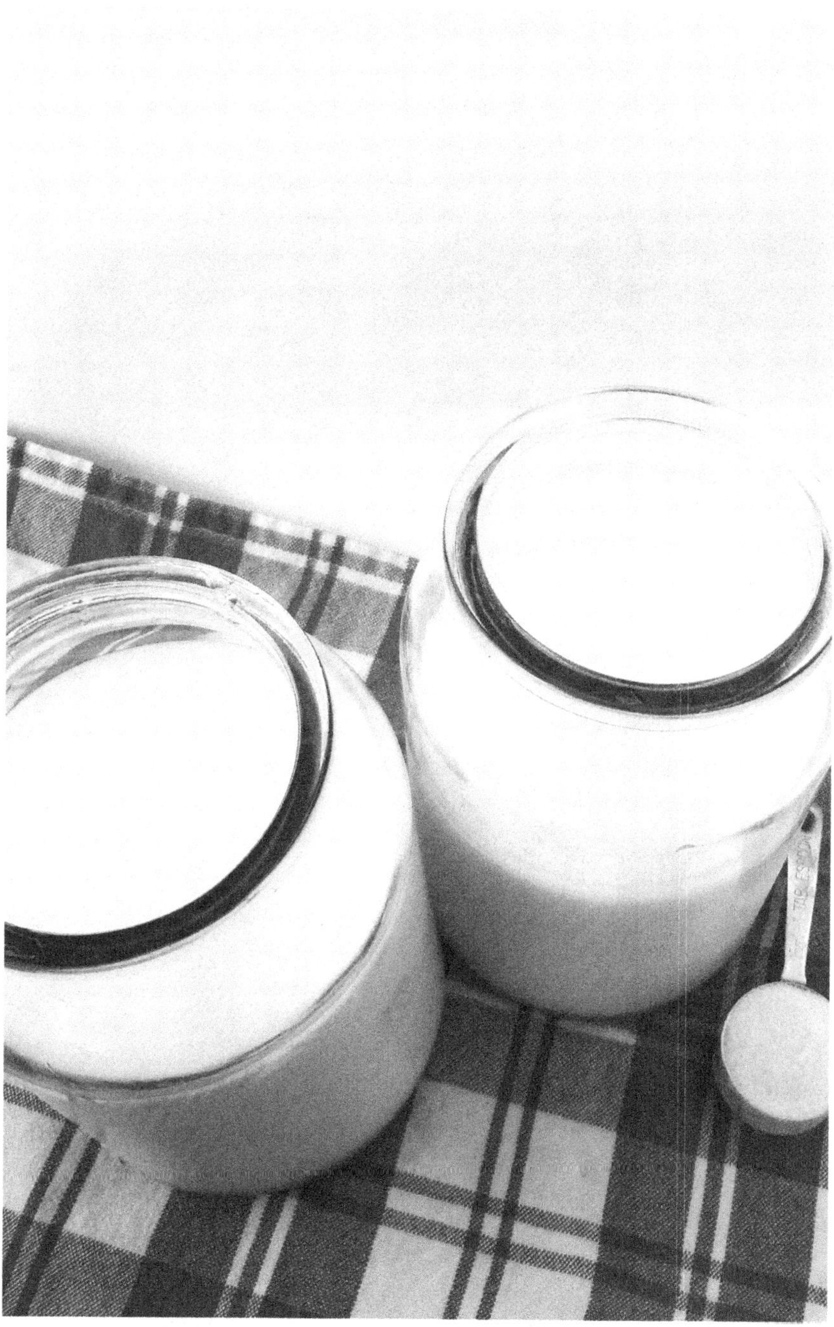

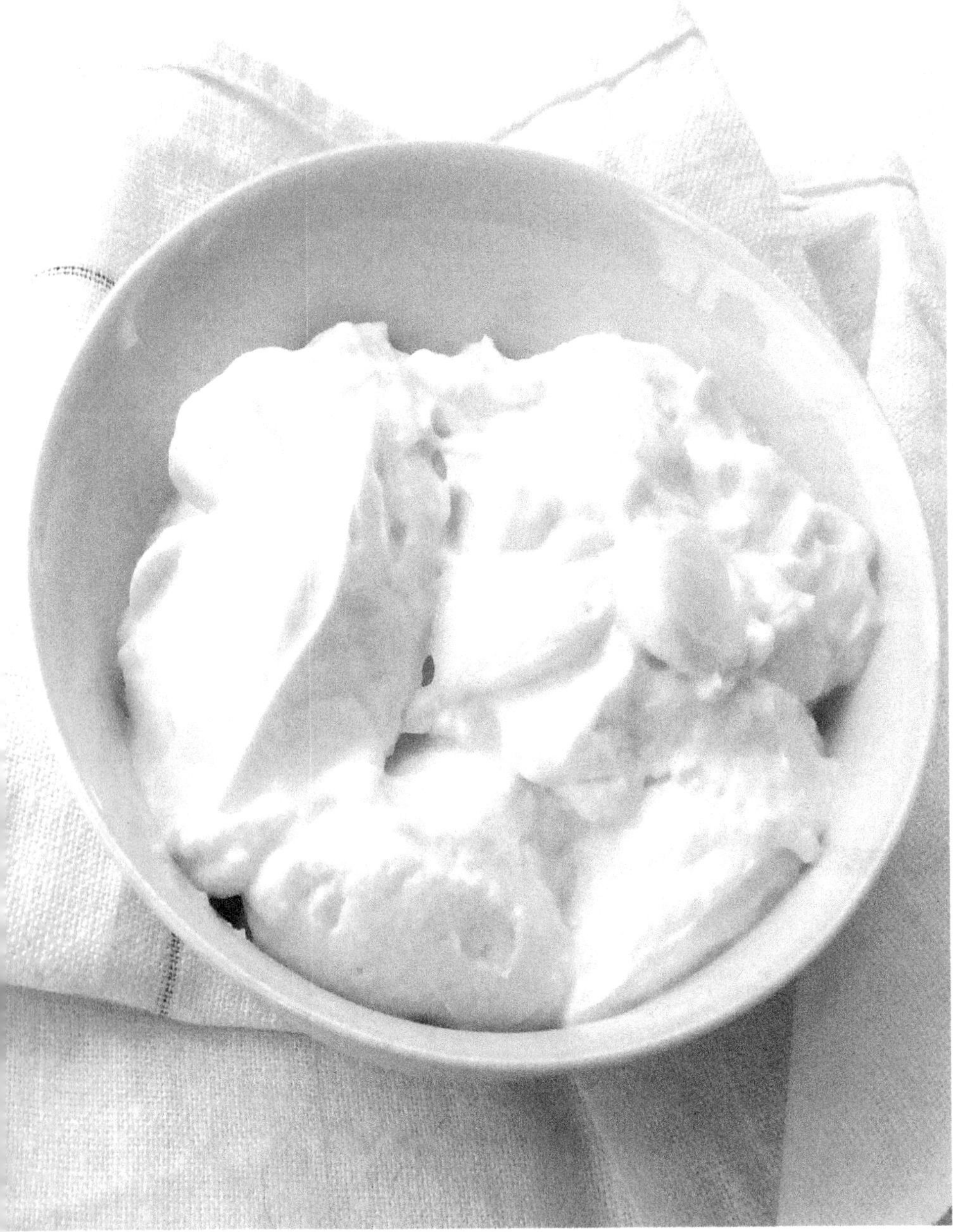

No Salt Ricotta Cheese

Homemade ricotta cheese is as cheap to make as the cost of a liter of milk. Homemade ricotta makes a great base for ravioli fillings and lasagna. You can serve with freshly sliced fruit: peaches, nectarines and berries. Or with stewed stone fruit: apricots, plums or fresh figs served with a drizzle of honey.

Makes: 2 cups
Cooking time: 30 minutes

Ingredients

8 cups whole milk

1 cup plain whole milk yogurt

1/2 cup heavy cream (optional for richer cheese)

2 tsp white wine vinegar or lemon juice

Method

Heat milk, yogurt and cream (if using) and vinegar in a heavy-bottomed saucepan.

Bring to boil on medium heat. Turn heat to low and boil very gently for 2 minutes, or until milk is curdled.

Remove from heat. Line a sieve or colander with 2 layers of clean cheesecloth or fine washed muslin. Set the colander into a deep bowl. Pour the milk mixture into the lined colander or sieve. Drain for 15 minutes. Pull sides of the cloth together and squeeze the curds gently to remove the whey (liquid). Remove strained curds from cloth and serve. You can store the ricotta cheese, in a covered container in the fridge for up to 3 days.

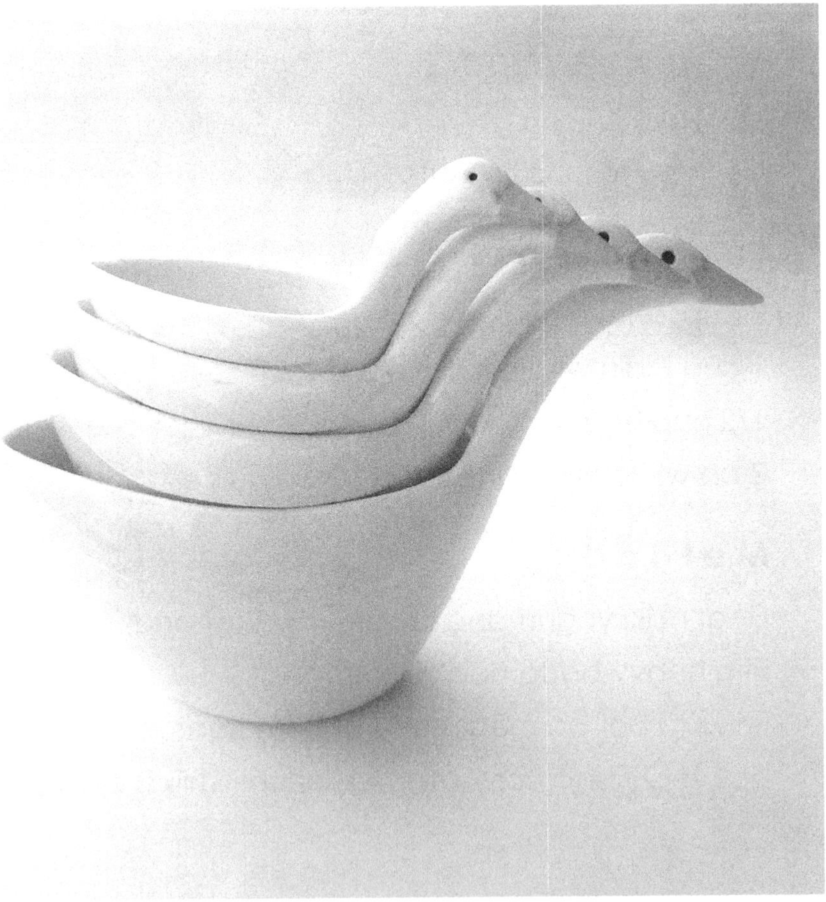

Yogurt Cheese

Makes: 2 cups plain yogurt

Method

Place yogurt in a cloth-lined sieve or a fine mesh strainer set over a bowl. Cover with cling film. Set aside at room temperature overnight.

Use instead of cottage cheese, sour cream. Add herbs and spices and use on crackers.

Crème Fraiche

Naturally soured fresh cream you can flavor with lemon zest, vanilla, or spices and use on top of fresh fruit for dessert.

Method

Stir 2 parts of fresh double cream with 1 part buttermilk, sour cream or yogurt (with live cultures). Stir over low heat until just warm. Allow to sit at room temperature for 6-8 hours. Stir and chill. Store covered in the fridge. Keeps for up to 3 weeks.

Homemade Buttermilk

Method

Add 1 tbsp lemon juice to 1 cup of milk. Mix well.

Pour into container and store in fridge.

Health Benefits Of Milk:
Good balance of protein, fat and carbohydrate. Important source of calcium, vitamin A, D, and B12.

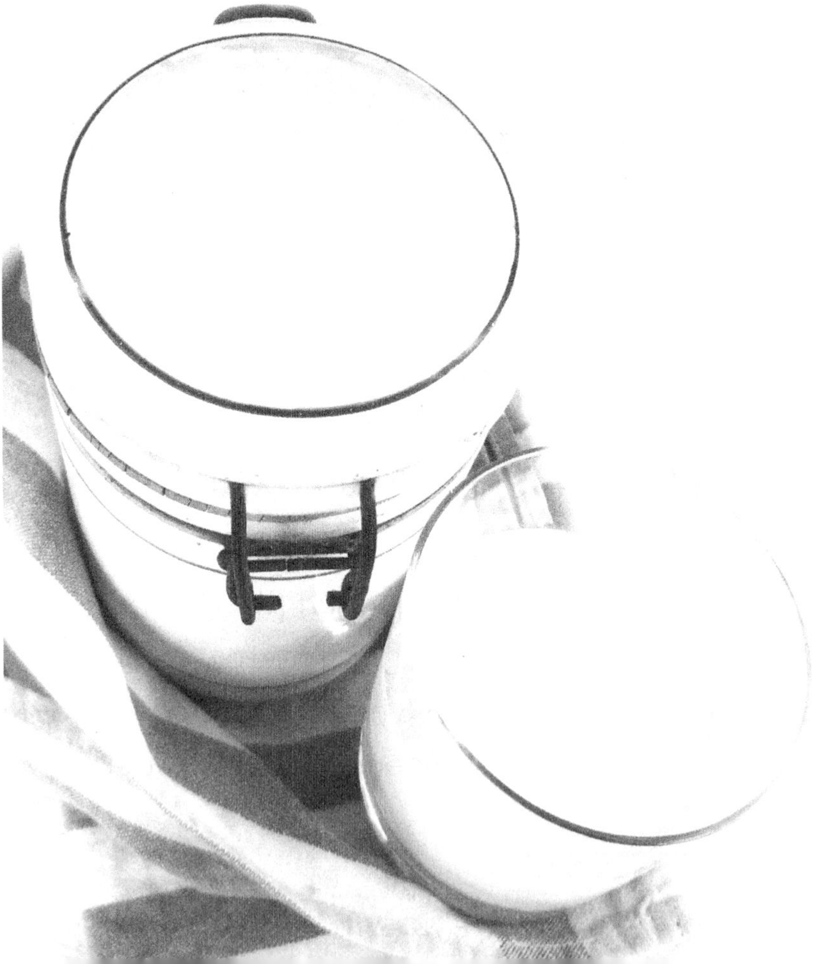

COOKING BASICS

Tomato Salsa

Ingredients

6 medium tomatoes

2 spring onions

30 ml (2 tbsp) lemon juice

1 tbsp parsley, chopped

10 cm length cucumber, diced

2 tbsp coriander

chopped bell-pepper (capsicum)

Method

Skin and seed tomatoes. Dice. Mix all ingredients together and chill 1-2 hours.

Serve with toasted pita bread chips.

Health Benefits Of Cucumber:
Rehydrates body and helps eliminate toxins. Good source of B vitamins for a quick-pick–me-up.

Mango Salsa

Ingredients

2 cups mango, cubed

1 onion, chopped

3 tbsp onion, chopped

3 tbsp oil

1 tbsp water

mint leaves or coriander leaves

fresh lime juice

Method

Place mango in a mixing bowl. Combine onion, oil and water in a saucepan. Cover and simmer on low heat for 10 minutes. Add mango. Add 1 tbsp fresh mint or coriander leaves. Stir in lime juice. Serve.

Health Benefits Of Mango:
Boost the immune system with generous levels of vitamin C, vitamin A and 25 kinds of carotenoids.

Dukkah

Ingredients

25g hazelnuts

25g almonds

1 tbsp smoked paprika

1 tbsp ground black pepper

3 tsp coriander seeds, roasted

2 tbsp thyme leaves

2 tsp garlic powder

Method

Roast nuts for 7-10 minutes. Put spices on a paper-lined baking sheet. Roast for 10 minutes, stirring frequently. Cool. Finely chop all in blender. Use as a healthy dip with yogurt; add to cooked vegetables; sprinkle over salad; coat potatoes before roasting; rub over meat or chicken before grilling or toss in cooked chickpeas for a salad.

Health Benefits Of Hazelnuts:
Rich in vitamin B complex. Helps the nervous system function and helps with stress, anxiety and depression.

Orange Oil

Combine 500ml strained orange juice and 50ml strained lemon juice into a saucepan. Reduce over low medium heat until syrup-like. Cool to room temperature then whisk in an equal quantity of olive oil. Store in clean bottles. Use to drizzle over grilled fish, potatoes, salads and steamed vegetables, such as asparagus and broccoli.

Prawn Oil

Take shells from prawns you peeled. Heat light olive oil in a frying pan. Add prawn heads and tails. Fry on low heat until prawns turn pink. Cook a further 20 minutes. Cool. Strain through kitchen paper. Discard shells. Pour oil into a clean bottle. Store in the fridge. Use when grilling fish or add with lime juice and black pepper to make a dressing for seafood salad or Asian noodle salad.

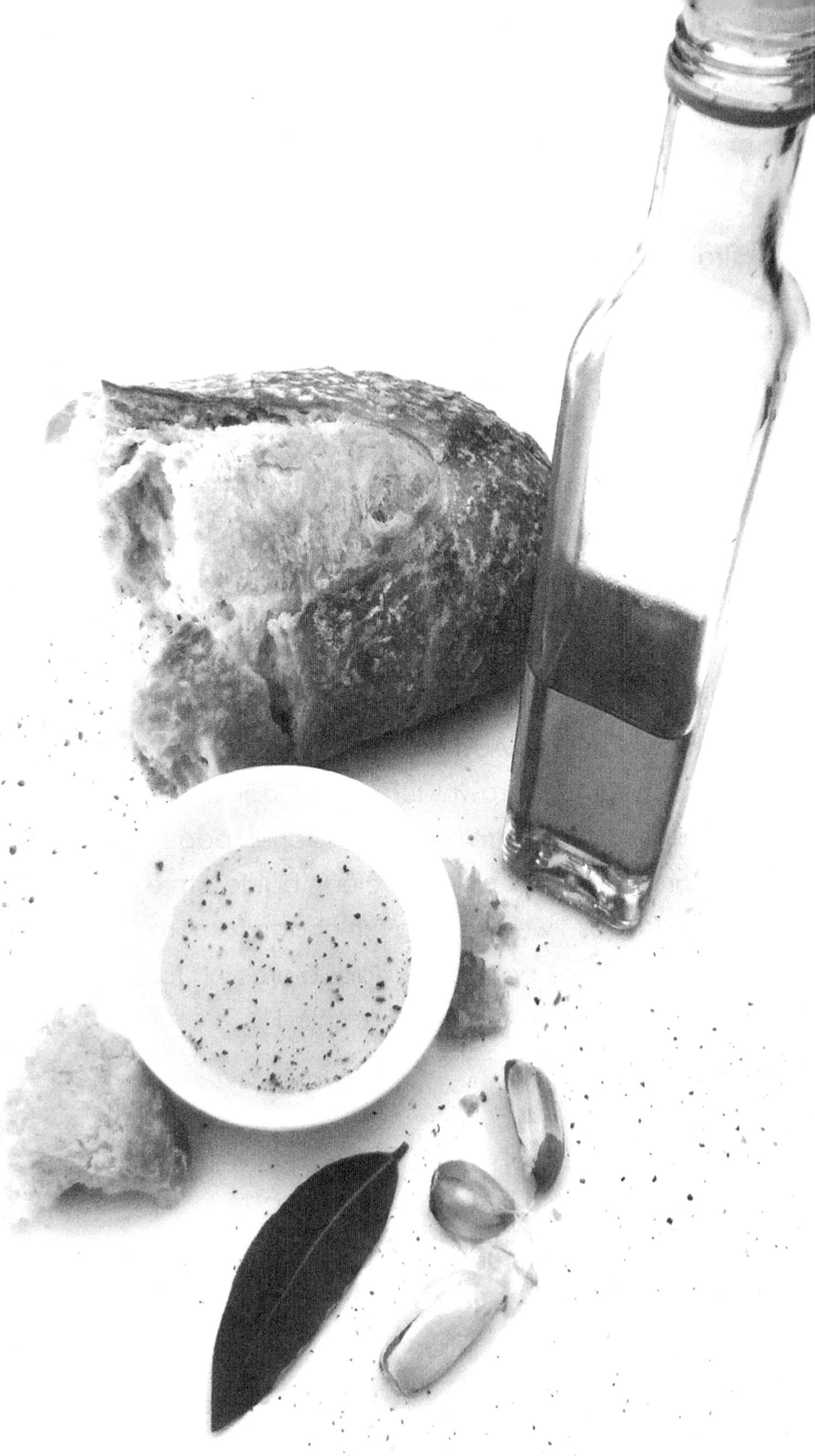

SALT SUBSTITUTES

The new salt is a garden of herbs.

Think of fresh herbs as 'the new salt'. There is an old Chinese saying, if you want to be happy all your life, plant a garden. I would add to that, plant a herb garden. Just a couple of pots or a planter box of herbs will make everything you cook taste so much better. Just a teaspoon of herbs can make food taste fresh and enlivened, giving depth and richness to stews, soups, casseroles and sauces. Seriously, there is nothing as wonderful as the scent of fresh basil. You can put the herbs in a shaker and use them at the table instead of salt. Use as a rub for meats and chicken. Add herbs to cooked vegetables. Add to sour cream for baked potatoes. Add to yogurt or soft cheeses for a tasty dip or dressing.

Rosemary, sage, oregano and marjoram are easy to grow. If they have enough sun, they will grow on a windowsill for months and you can use them everyday.

Seasonal herbs, like basil, parsley, coriander and chervil need regular cutting and in particular you must keep the flower or seed heads from forming. When you trim these, the plants will keep growing until late season.

You can use fresh herbs from your garden or bought from the store and then dry them in a low oven turned off, overnight. Fill glass pantry jars, and small tins with herb seasonings, and add zest to everything you cook. Herb blends enhance foods such as fish, chicken, beef, vegetables. Piquant blends such as dill, savory, thyme and garlic can help you eliminate salt without loss or favor or taste. Here are easy to make special blends.

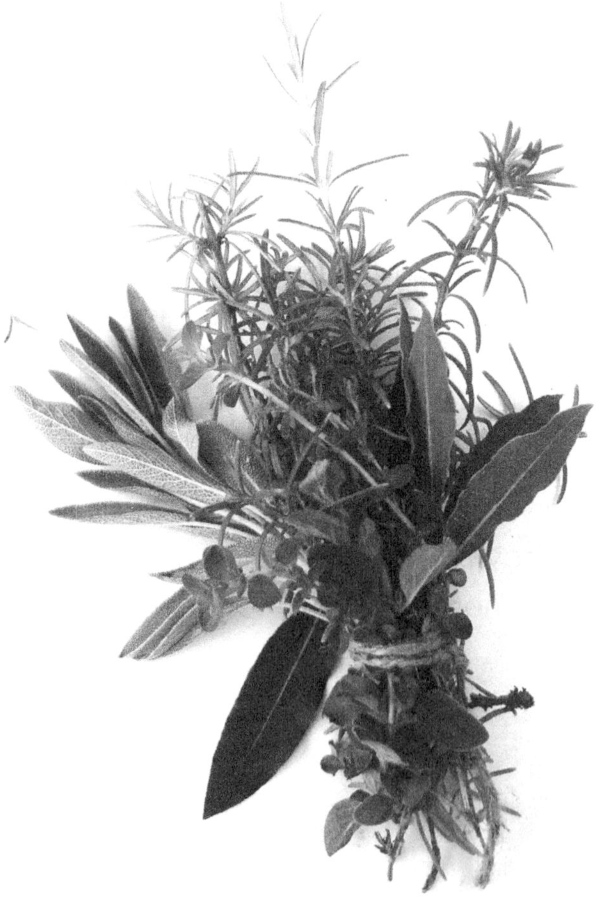

French Blend

Makes: 1/3 cup

Ingredients

2 tbsp dried dill

2 tbsp dried chives

1 tbsp dried oregano

2 tsp celery seeds

1/2 tsp ground black pepper

Method

Place ingredients into a blender. Process until the herbs are well mixed together.

Spice Island Blend

Makes: 1/3 cup

Ingredients

1 tbsp ground cloves

1 tbsp cracked black pepper

1 tbsp crushed coriander seeds

1/2 tsp garlic powder

Method

Mix together and store in a cool place.

Moroccan Blend

Ingredients

3 tbsp ground cinnamon

1 1/2 tbsp ground black pepper

1 1/2 tbsp ground white pepper

2 1/2 tsp ground nutmeg

2 1/2 tsp ground cloves

2 1/2 tsp ground cardamom

Method

Mix together and store in a cool place.

Chicken Herbs

Ingredients

1 tbsp dried marjoram

2 tbsp dried tarragon

1 tbsp dried basil

1 tbsp dried rosemary

1 tsp paprika

Mix well and store in a jar.

Fish Herbs

Ingredients

3 tbsp dill

2 tbsp dried basil

1 tbsp dried tarragon

1 tbsp lemon thyme

1 tbsp dried parsley

1 tbsp dried chervil

Mix well and store in a jar.

Pork Herbs

Ingredients

3 tbsp ground coriander

2 tbsp ground cumin

1 tbsp ground ginger

2 tbsp dried sage

1 tbsp dried thyme

Mix well and store in a jar.

Fine Herbs

Ingredients

2 tbsp dried chervil

2 tbsp dried chives

2 tbsp dried tarragon

2 tbsp dried parsley

Mix well and store in a jar.

Bouquet Garni

Ingredients

1/4 cup dried parsley leaves

4 bay leaves crumbled

2 tbsp dried thyme

2 tbsp dried marjoram

Method

Mix herbs together. Place 1 teaspoon in a small muslin bag or 6 cm square of cheesecloth doubled. Tie bag or gather up the corners and tie with kitchen string. Use in soups, stews and stocks.

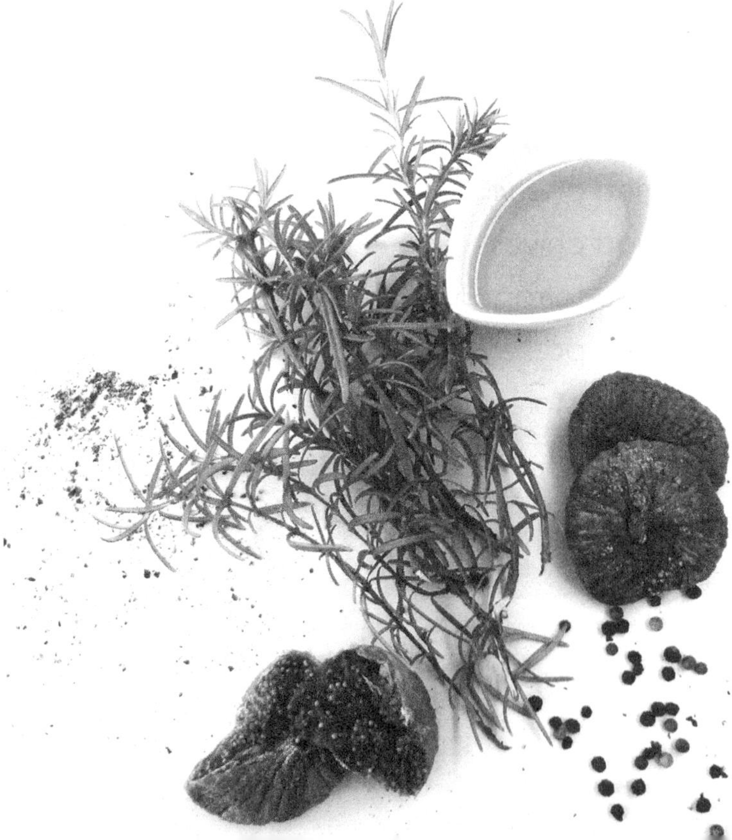

Italian Seasoning

Use on pizzas, pasta, herb bread, or any dish that needs Italian flavor.

Ingredients

1/2 cup dried oregano

1/2 cup dried basil

1/4 cup dried parsley

1 tbsp fennel seeds, crushed

2 tbsp dried sage

1 tbsp red pepper flakes

Mix well and store in a jar.

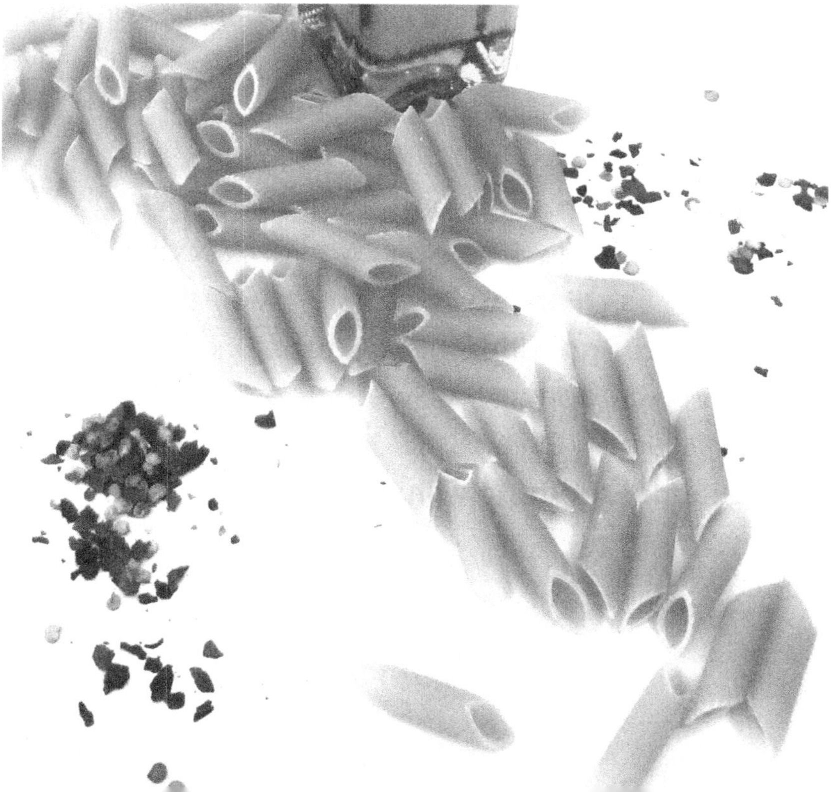

INGREDIENT KNOW HOW

What goes with what?

Follow your instincts. Substitute one ingredient for another. Use other ingredients on hand, when you don't have exactly the right ingredients. The dish will be slightly different but still taste good. For example, if you don't have spinach, use rocket. If you don't have beans, use asparagus. If you don't have shallots, use red onion.

Basil goes with: Eggplants, Tomatoes, Olive oil, Lamb, Potatoes, Pine Nuts, Walnuts, Zucchini, Capsicum, Fish, Prawns, Pasta.

Bay leaves go with: Stocks, Soups, Dried beans, Lentils, Broad beans, Pork, Sweet peppers, Veal, Potatoes, Garlic, Onions, Milk

Coriander seeds go with: Beef, Lamb, Lentils,

Mushrooms, Chickpeas, Eggplants, Chicken, Hazelnuts.

Chives go with: Chicken, Eggs, Fish, Potatoes, Cucumber, Celery, Beetroot, Butter, Eggs, Prawns, Fish, Beef, Shallots, Garlic, Pork,

Coriander leaves go with: Prawns, Garlic, Pork, Beef, Avocado, Fish, Ginger, Coconut, Noodles, Soup, Mint, Parsley, Chicken, Yogurt

Fennel goes with: Olive oil, Lemon juice, Pepper, Chicken stock, Pasta, Olive oil, Tomatoes, Almonds, Walnuts, Fish, Garlic, Mushrooms, Chicken, Potatoes, Eggs, Rocket, Watercress,

Garlic goes with: Potatoes, Butter, Olive oil, Lamb, Pork, Veal, Fish, Shellfish, Basil, Rosemary, Fennel, Parsley, Spinach, Saffron, Eggs

Ginger goes with: Nutmeg, Raisins, Honey, Cinnamon, Cardamom, Almonds, Cloves, Brown sugar, Aniseed

Honey goes with: Cream, Fruit, Dried Fruit, Cardamom, Cinnamon, Nuts, Chicken, Pork, Ginger, Cloves, Dried beans

Lemons go with: Fish, Veal, Chicken, Shellfish, Fish, Cream, Eggs, Oranges, Honey, Tea, Pasta, Noodles, Rice, Raspberries, Papaya, Coriander, Cumin Seed

Mint goes with: Lamb, Potatoes, Peas, Carrots, Tea, Lime juice, Garlic, Noodles, Bean sprouts, Pork, Cucumbers, Parsley, Coriander, Cracked wheat,

Oregano goes with: Tomatoes, Eggs, Dried Beans,

Rice, Grilled fish, Lamb, Sweet Corn, Sweet peppers, Chicken, Lemons, Eggplant

Parsley goes with: Butter, Garlic, Pepper, Fish, Cream, Pepper, Lemon juice, Pine Nuts, Beans, Eggs, Lentils, Chickpeas, Chives, Chervil, Tarragon, Olive oil, Pasta, Zucchini, Artichokes, Mint, Cumin, Radishes

Rosemary goes with: Lamb, Pork, Chicken, Potatoes, Bread, Olive oil, Garlic, Parsley, Onions, Tomatoes, Yogurt, Fish, Pine nuts

Sage goes with: Butter, Pumpkin, Olive oil, Veal, Chicken, Potatoes, Sweet potato, Pasta, Duck, Lamb, Lemons, Dried beans, Peas, Onions, Leeks

Salad greens go with: Potato, Pumpkin, Eggplant, Sweet Pepper, Beetroot, Onion, Garlic, Green Beans, Dried Beans, Asparagus, Artichoke, Chickpeas, Carrot, Broccoli, Prawns, Squid, Poultry, Egg

Tarragon goes with: Chicken, Fish, Egg, Shallot, Beef, Tomatoes, Mayonnaise

Vinegar goes with: Salad Greens, Cucumber, Strawberries, Peppercorns, Herbs, Fish, Olive oil

Almonds go with: Honey, Peach, Apricot, Vanilla, Cream, Chicken

Cashews go with: Coconut milk Beans, Cauliflower, Fish, Chicken, Almond, Rice

Coconut goes with: Chicken, Fish, Beef, Rice, Turmeric, Kaffir Lime, Lemongrass

Hazelnuts go with: Almond, Pork, Duck, Cinnamon, Orange

Peanuts go with: Pork, Chicken, Beef, Cucumber, Beans

Pecans go with: Garlic, Maple Syrup, Lemon Juice, Molasses, Pine nuts, Basil, Veal, Pasta, Garlic, Rice, Salad, Lime

Pistachios go with: Rice, Yogurt, Honey, Semolina, Almond, Walnut, Pears, Garlic, Cream

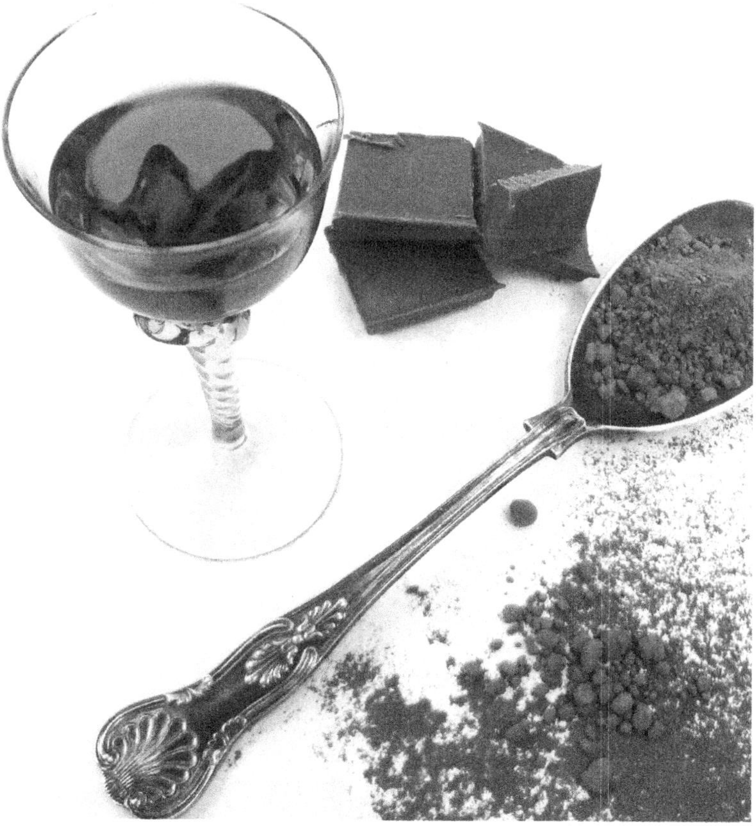

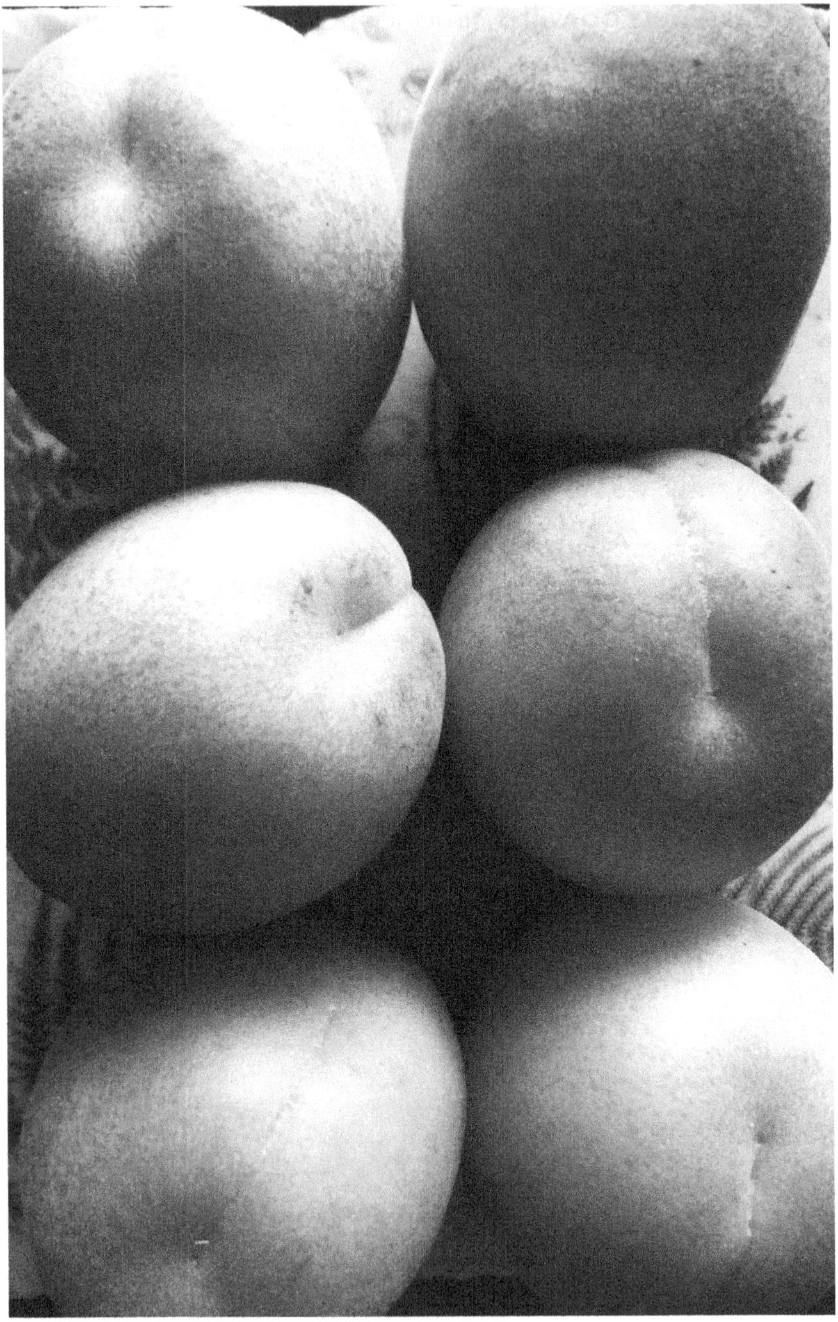

BREAKFAST

Breakfast is an important meal. Your body needs a big boost every morning to raise your metabolic rate and give you energy for the day. When you have Meniere's, the best thing you can do for yourself, is to eat breakfast before starting your day. No computer, no phone calls...until after you've eaten. Complex carbohydrates found in whole grains supply fiber and convert easily to glucose, fueling your system. Protein keeps you going.

Angel In The Morning

Smoothies boost your vitamin intake for the day.

Serves: 2-3

Ingredients

2 cups fresh or frozen fruit (banana, berries)

1 cup plain yogurt (to taste)

1 cup water

1-2 tbsp honey

1/2 cup fruit juice (apple, orange) or milk

Method

Place into blender. Blend until smooth.

Health Benefits Of Bananas:
High in potassium to protect the heart. Contains a natural mood-enhancer, tryptophan. Now you know why monkeys are so happy!

Very Berry Smoothie

Full of antioxidants and vitamins. Whip up this smoothie and load up on nutrients.

Serves: 4

Ingredients

4 cups water or coconut water

1 cup frozen blueberries

1 banana

1 tbsp virgin coconut oil

15 almonds

1 tsp ground cinnamon

5 tbsp shredded coconut

2 tbsp honey

1 tbsp spirulina powder (optional)

Method

Place ingredients in blender. Blend for 2 minutes on high. Pour into glasses and serve.

Health Benefits Of Blueberries:
These berries rank 31st in antioxidant activity compared with 60 other fruits. High in vitamin A and potassium.

Banana Apple Smoothie

Serves: 2

Ingredients

1 banana

1 cup frozen raspberries

1 cup apple juice

1/2 tsp honey

Method

Place in a blender. Blend until smooth.

Health Benefits Of Raspberries:
High in foliate and magnesium.

Raw Energy Juice

Serves: 4

Ingredients

1 raw beetroot, peeled, cut in chunks

2 carrots, peeled

3 apples, cored

1 stalk celery, washed

2 cm piece fresh ginger, peeled

Method

Put vegetables through a juicer. Pour into glasses and serve immediately.

Health Benefits Of Apples:
Apples are rich in antioxidants.

Buttermilk Pancakes

Makes: 16

250g (2 cups) organic plain flour
2 tsp baking powder
2 tbsp sugar
2 eggs lightly beaten
3 cups buttermilk
75g
unsalted butter, melted and cooled
unsalted butter for cooking

Method

Mix flour, baking powder and sugar together. Whisk eggs, melted butter and buttermilk together. Stir into flour and whisk together until smooth. Heat frying pan over medium heat. Add a knob of butter. Melt butter. Spoon 1/3 cup pancake mixture for each pancake into pan. Cook until one side bubbles. Flip over. Cook for another minute until golden. Serve pancakes with stewed or fresh fruit, maple syrup and plain yogurt.

French Toast

Serves: 4

Ingredients

8 slices of brioche or French bread, sliced thickly
3 large free-range eggs
3/4 cup (185 ml) milk
30g unsalted butter
berries (strawberries, raspberries, blueberries). Fresh or frozen (thawed).

Method

Place eggs and milk in a bowl. Whisk together. Dip brioche or bread into the mixture until soaked through. Heat a little of the butter in a frying pan over medium heat to grease pan. Add bread pieces. Cook for 1 minute on each side until golden. Sprinkle with a dusting of icing sugar (confectioners sugar). Serve with berry sauce.

Berry Sauce: Place 2 cups berries in a blender with 1/4 cup (60g) caster sugar and 1 tbsp lemon or lime juice. Blend together.

Breakfast Compote

Make this up and store covered in the fridge.

Serves: 6-8

Ingredients

1 cup dried figs

500 ml apple juice

2 cups water

1/2 cup raw sugar

3 cinnamon sticks

10 whole cloves

10 peppercorns

4 green cardamom pods, crushed

1 vanilla bean, split in half lengthwise

rind of 1 lemon or lime cut in thin strips

1 cup dark raisins

6 fresh pears (or apples) peeled

Method

Soak figs in water for 2 hours. Drain. Set aside.

In a saucepan, combine fruit juice, water, sugar,

cinnamon, peppercorns, vanilla bean, cloves and lemon rind. Simmer for 15 minutes on low heat. Add dried fruits. Simmer for a further 10 minutes. Using a slotted spoon, remove the fruits and place in a bowl. Add pears or (apples) and poach in the same saucepan for 8 minutes, until cooked but firm. Add dried fruits back to the pan. Cool to room temperature. Place in a serving bowl. Serve at room temperature or chilled, with plain yogurt.

Noah's Pancakes

Ingredients

2 cups (organic) plain flour
2 eggs
2 egg yolks
2 cups milk
2 tbsp unsalted butter, melted

Method

Place all ingredients in a blender. Blend until smooth. Or place in a bowl and whisk together. Heat butter in a crepe pan or small frying pan. Add pancake batter. Roll around the pan to coat thinly. These are traditional French crepe style (not thick). Cook on medium heat a few minutes. Flip over and cook the other side. Remove from pan. Keep warm in a low oven. Repeat until you have a stack of pancakes. Serve with your choice of maple syrup, berries, bananas, honey, or with a squeeze of lime or lemon and a little caster sugar.

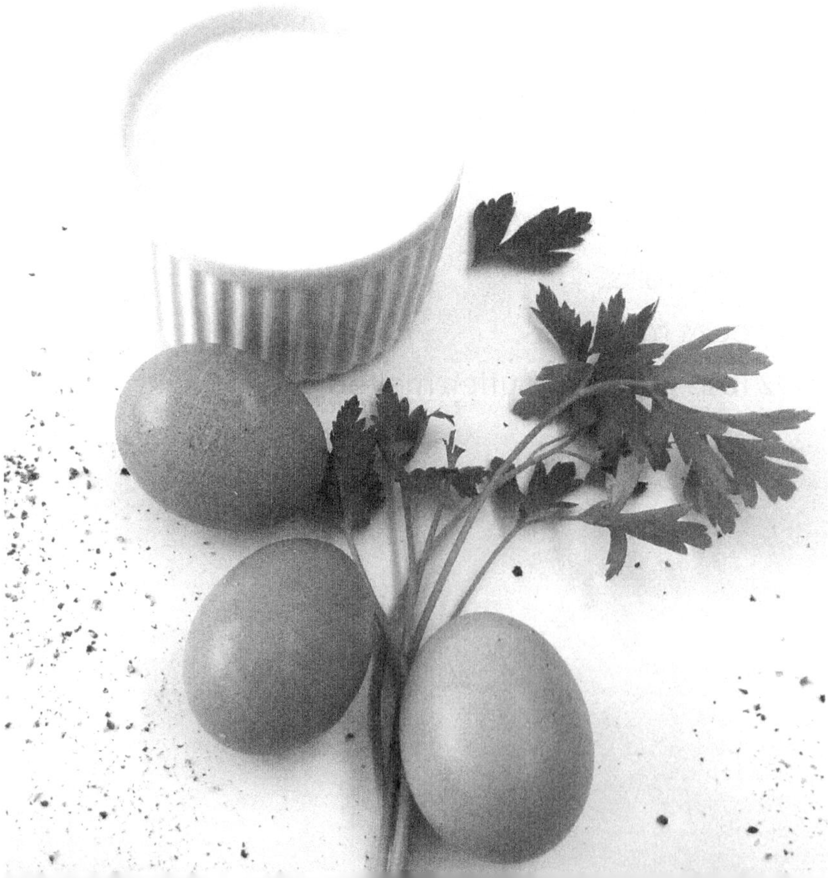

Hash Brown Pancakes

Serves: 4-6

Ingredients

3 large potatoes

1 tbsp finely chopped onion

1 egg, beaten

freshly ground black pepper

1 tbsp olive oil

2 tbsp olive oil for frying

Method

Peel potatoes. Grate them and squeeze out excess water with your hands. Add onion and egg. Let mixture stand for 2 minutes. Squeeze out any excess moisture. Heat oil in a frying pan. When oil is hot, spoon in tablespoons of the potato mixture. Flatten each with a fork to form a small pancake. Fry on both sides until golden brown. Drain on kitchen paper. Serve hot.

Italian Sausages

Makes: 12

Ingredients

1 kg minced chicken/veal

1 medium onion, roughly chopped

1/2 cup flat-leaf parsley, finely chopped

2 tbsp fresh sage, finely chopped

6 cloves garlic, finely minced

1 tsp ground fennel seeds

1/2 tsp ground cloves

1 tsp ground black pepper

Method

Combine ingredients in a mixing bowl. Mix well. Form into 6 sausages. Roll in a little flour to dust. Set aside in the fridge for 1 hour before cooking. Heat a frying pan with a little oil. Place sausages into the pan. Cook over medium heat until brown.

Health Benefits Of Parsley:
Rich in vitamin C, B12, K and A. Heals the nervous system.

Baked Beans

Serves: 4-6

Ingredients

1 tbsp olive oil
1 onion, finely chopped
1 clove garlic
1 tsp fresh thyme leaves, finely chopped
1/2 tsp dried oregano
400g tinned tomatoes
2 x 400g tins no salt added cannellini (white) beans, rinsed and drained, or use 800g dried beans, soaked, cooked, then drained.
freshly ground black pepper

Method

Heat oven to 160 C. Place oil in a casserole dish. Heat over medium heat. Add onions. Cook until transparent. Add garlic, thyme, oregano and cook for 1 minute. Add tomatoes and 1/2 cup water. Bring to boil on medium heat. Reduce heat. Simmer 10 minutes. Remove from heat. Place lid on casserole. Bake in oven for 25 minutes. Serve.

Toasted Muesli

Ingredients

300g (3 cups) organic rolled oats

125 ml (1/2 cup) apple juice

2 tbsp light olive oil

1/2 cup almonds (with skins on)

1 cup sunflower seeds

1/4 cup pepitas (pumpkin seeds)

1/2 cup flaked coconut

1 cup dried blueberries, cranberries, or raisins

Method

Heat oven to 160 C. Place ingredients in a bowl, except the dried berries. Spread over an oven tray in one layer. Bake 25-30 minutes, until golden brown. Turn the mixture over while baking to cook evenly. Remove from heat. Add dried fruit. Cool. Place in a covered container in the fridge. Keeps up to 1 month. To serve, place in serving bowls. Add milk, yogurt and serve with fresh berries or grated apple and a dusting of cinnamon.

Toasted Wheat Germ Muesli

Serves: 30

Ingredients

750g rolled oats

250g barley flakes

1/2 cup roasted buckwheat

1/3 cup sesame seeds

1 cup wheat germ

1 cup coconut flakes

1 cup flaked almonds

250g dried fruits, chopped

1/2 cup pumpkin seeds

1/2 cup sunflower seeds

Method

Place oats on an oven tray and bake in a moderate oven for 5-10 minutes, until golden. Cool. Toast coconut, sesame seeds, and almonds in a dry frying pan. Stir to prevent burning. Cool. Mix all ingredients together and add chopped dried fruits. Store in an airtight container for up to one month.

Swiss Muesli

Serves: 4-6

Ingredients

1 cup organic rolled oats

1/2 cup barley flakes

3/4 cup milk

1 apple, cored, grated with skin

1 punnet fresh blueberries (or use 1 extra apple)

1 tbsp honey

1/2 cup plain yogurt

1/4 cup almond flakes, toasted

1/2 tsp cinnamon

Method

Mix oats and barley with milk. Refrigerate overnight. Next morning add the other ingredients and serve.

Health Benefits Of Barley:
Good source of vitamin B1, chromium, magnesium, zinc.

Quinoa Berry Porridge

Ingredients

Per person

100g quinoa

200 ml water

50 ml organic or coconut milk

1 tsp cinnamon

50gm berries

Method

Wash quinoa in sieve. Place in pot with water. Bring to boil; allow to simmer (with lid on). After 15 minutes water should have almost evaporated. Remove lid to allow to evaporate completely. Add milk, cinnamon and berries. Stir for a few minutes to allow milk to soak up. Add yogurt or more milk to taste. You can make a big batch and keep in the fridge and then warm up with some milk in the morning. Keeps for two days.

Health Benefits Of Quinoa:
Protein rich. Contains 9 essential amino acids. This grain was "the gold of the Incas".

Fruit Muesli

Ingredients

200g (2 cups) organic rolled oats

1 cup water

2 tbsp organic stabilized wheat germ

2 tbsp honey

2 tbsp toasted hazelnuts or almonds, chopped

1 apple, grated with skin on

1 cup orange, pear or apple juice

1/2 tsp cinnamon

1/2 cup yogurt

Method

Soak rolled oats in water overnight. Add yogurt, honey, wheat germ and nuts. Top with grated apple and a dusting of powdered cinnamon. Instead of apple use any fresh fruit, cut in chunks, e.g. nectarines, peaches, apricots, oranges, berries or banana.

Health Benefits Of Oats:
High in fiber and a good source of essential vitamins. Contains beta glucan, which speeds up the body's response to infection and helps with faster healing.

Secret Muesli

Ingredients

3 cups rolled oats

1 cup rye flakes

1 cup oat bran

1/2 cup pumpkin seeds

1/2 cup sunflower seeds

1/2 cup wheat germ

1/2 cup almonds

1/4 cup sesame seeds

1/2 cup shredded coconut

3 cups mixed dried fruits e.g. apricots, raisins, apple, ginger

1 tsp grated nutmeg

1-2 tsp cinnamon

Method

Combine all ingredients together. Store in sealed containers in the fridge. Use as a dry muesli served with yogurt, fruit and honey. Or serve as moist muesli. For moist muesli, soak 2 cups of dry muesli in a cup of water overnight in the fridge. Mix with 1/2 cup of natural yogurt, 2 tbsp freshly chopped almonds and top with grated apple or your choice of fresh fruit.

Health Benefits Of Rye:
Supplies high levels of iron, calcium, potassium and zinc. Helps to balance blood sugar levels.

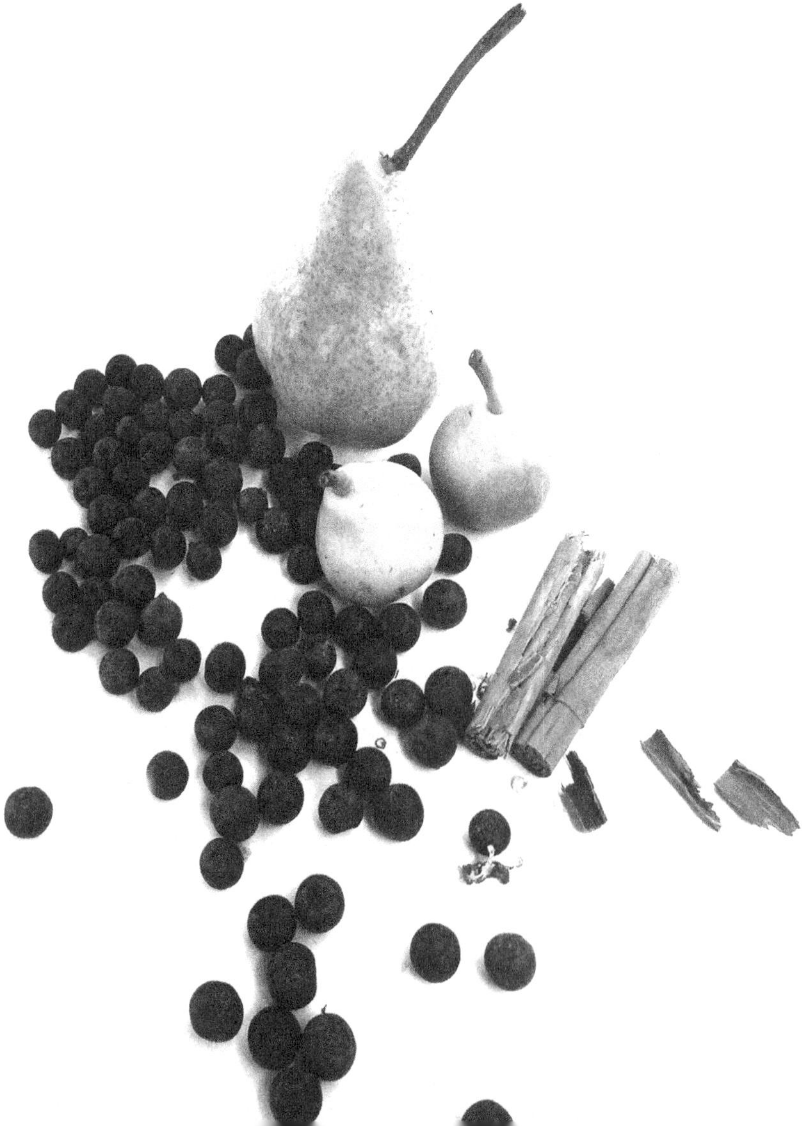

Baked Granola

Ingredients

2 cups raw organic oats

1/2 cup sunflower seeds

1 tsp ground cinnamon

3 tsp honey

100 ml mild olive oil

2 tsp pure vanilla extract

1/4 cup slivered almonds

1/4 cup pine nuts

dried berries (blueberries, cranberries or dried cherries) to add at the end of cooking.

Method

Heat oven to 160 C. Place dry ingredients in a large bowl. Add honey, oil, vanilla and mix well. Spread onto a baking tray. Bake 10 minutes. Turn over. Bake a further 10 minutes. Remove from oven. Stir in dried berries. Cool. Place into airtight container. Keeps 2 weeks in the fridge or in freeze for up to 3 months.

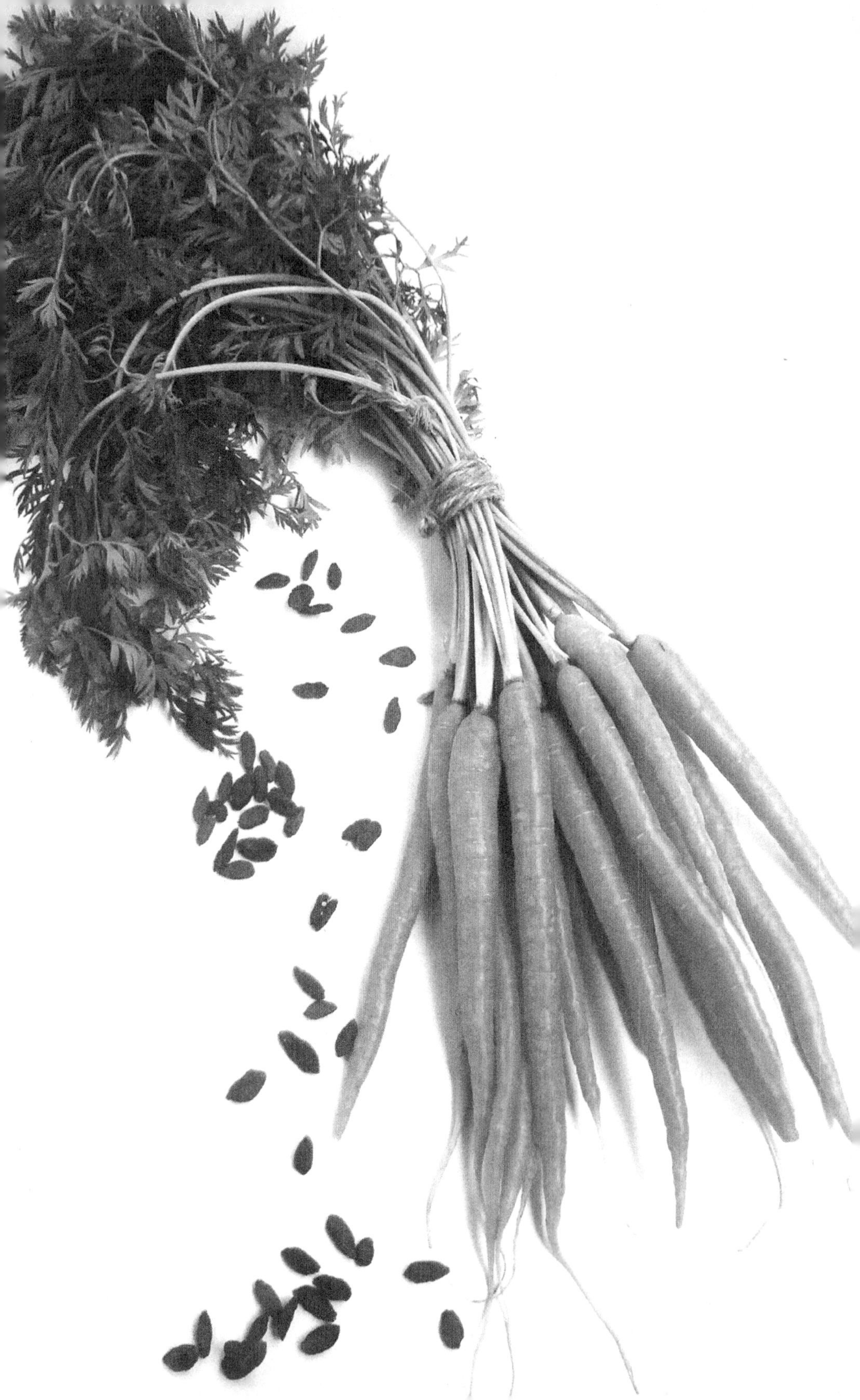

SOUPS AND STOCKS

Chicken Stock Without Salt

Ingredients

6 parsley stalks, finely chopped

2 sprigs of fresh thyme, or pinch of dried thyme

1 bay leaf

6 peppercorns

1.5 liters cold water

1 whole chicken

250ml white wine or water

50g butter

2 leeks (white part only) finely chopped

1/2 carrot, finely chopped

1 stick celery, finely chopped

1 clove garlic, finely chopped

1 small onion, finely chopped

Method

Melt butter in a saucepan. Add leek, celery, carrot, garlic and onion. Cook over low heat until the vegetables become transparent and soft. Add the whole chicken, turning it in the vegetables. Add herbs and peppercorns. Add 250ml of water or wine. Place lid on the pot. Steam chicken over high heat for 5 minutes. Add the cold water and bring to a slow simmer. Simmer for 1 hour.

Cool chicken and remove meat and skin. Place bones back into the pot. Simmer for another hour. Strain bones through a fine sieve. Cool. Place in fridge overnight. Remove any fat. Store in the fridge or freezer.

Poached chicken can be used in recipes such as salads, pasta and sandwiches.

Health Benefits Of Chicken:
Contains B5, which has a calming effect on the nerves. Trace minerals boost the immune system. Contains zinc and calcium.

Beef Stock

Ingredients

1.5 kg beef marrow bones

2 large carrots

2 onions, quartered

3 stalks celery, cut in chunks

2.25 liters cold water

2 parsley stalks

1 bay leaf

8 black peppercorns

1/2 tsp dried thyme

Method

Heat oven to 230 C (450 F)

Place bones, carrot, onions and celery in a roasting pan. Place in oven and roast for 40 minutes. Remove from oven and place bones and vegetables into a large saucepan. Place 2 cups of the water in the roasting pan and cook on medium heat, stirring the brownings off the bottom. Remove from heat and pour over the bones. Add the rest of the water, parsley, peppercorns and thyme.

Bring to boil on high heat. Skim off scum and

discard. Lower heat, cover pan with lid and simmer gently for 4 hours. Cool. Strain through a sieve. Place in the fridge covered overnight. Remove congealed fat. Stock is ready to use or freeze in batches for later use.

Potassium Rich Vegetable Stock

Use as a base for soups, sauces or in stews to replace water or wine.

Serves 6

1 cup onion, chopped
1 carrot, coarsely chopped
1 cup celery, coarsely chopped
1 whole head garlic, skins removed
2 strips lemon peel
2 bay leaves
2 sprigs thyme
1 tbsp oregano

5 sprigs flat-leaf parsley
10 peppercorns
1 small cinnamon stick
olive oil

Method

Place a little olive oil in a stock pan. Heat on medium. Add vegetables. Cook for 10 minutes until the onions become transparent. Take care not to brown. Reduce heat. Cover vegetables with water. Bring to boil. Reduce heat to simmer. Cover pan and simmer for 40 minutes. Remove from heat. Cool. Strain broth through a sieve. Store in covered containers in the freezer or fridge.

Health Benefits Of Celery:
Celery contains super nutrients including magnesium. Soothes the nervous system. Promotes restful sleep.

Tomato And Saffron Soup

An exotic fresh tasting soup with a deliciously complex flavor.

Ingredients

1 onion, finely sliced

2 leeks, white part only, finely sliced

6 cloves garlic, crushed

8 large ripe tomatoes, chopped

1 heaped tsp saffron stamens

1 sprig fresh thyme

1 sprig fresh marjoram or oregano

500 ml chicken stock

1 tbsp tomato paste

freshly ground black pepper

Method

Heat a little olive oil. Add onions, garlic and leeks. Cook until soft and transparent. Add tomatoes, saffron, thyme, oregano and saffron. Add chicken stock. Simmer on low heat for 20 minutes. Add tomato paste to taste. Stir. Simmer 5 minutes on low heat. Season with pepper. Cool. Place in food processor or blender and process until smooth. Reheat and serve.

Leek And Potato Soup

Serves: 4-6

Ingredients

4 leeks (white part only)

2 large potatoes, peeled and diced

1 onion, finely chopped

50g butter

900 ml chicken stock

275 ml milk

freshly ground white or black pepper

2 tbsp chopped parsley or chives for garnish

Method

Cut off the green top and tough outer layer of the leeks. Split the stalks and clean well to remove any earth. Cut them finely. Drain.

Place butter in a heavy saucepan. Add leeks, onion and potatoes. Stir well. Cover and cook on a low heat for 10 minutes. Add stock and milk. Stir well. Bring to a simmer. Place lid on the pan. Cook gently for about 20 minutes, stirring frequently. Remove from heat. Cool. Place in a blender and puree. Return to pan. Add freshly ground pepper. Place in a serving bowl or individual bowls. Add garnish. You can serve this soup hot or chilled. Chilled potato and leek soup is called Vichyssoise.

Health Benefits Of Leeks:

Helps insomnia and anxiety. A good source of vitamin A, vitamin B6 and vitamin C. Contains antioxidant properties and protects blood vessels.

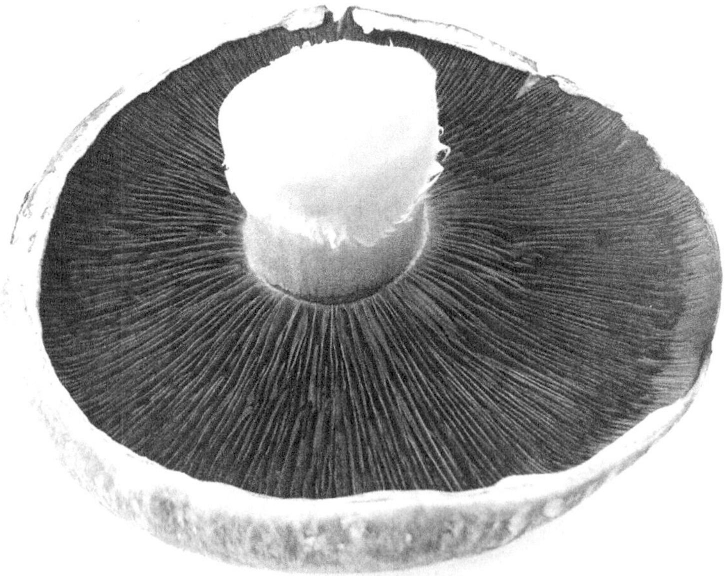

Mushroom Soup

Ingredients

350g Portobello or brown mushrooms
2 large potatoes, peeled and chopped
25g unsalted butter
2 cloves garlic, finely chopped
freshly ground black pepper
1 tsp finely chopped fresh oregano
6 cups homemade chicken stock
1/2 cup milk or thin cream

Method

Wash mushrooms. Chop. Heat butter in a large saucepan. Add garlic and mushrooms. Cook on medium heat for 10 minutes. Add potatoes, stock and oregano. Bring to the boil on medium heat. Reduce heat to low and simmer for 20 minutes. Cool to room temperature. Place soup in a blender in small batches. Place blended soup back in the saucepan. Add milk or cream very slowly while heat is on low. Do not boil. Serve in a soup tureen or in individual bowls. Garnish with parsley. Serve with toasted garlic bread.

Spinach And Ginger Soup

Ingredients

2 leeks, white part only, sliced

50 ml olive oil

4 cloves garlic

40g fresh ginger root, to taste

1.5 liters chicken stock

500g English spinach, washed, stalks removed

ground black pepper to taste

Method

Place oil in a pan. Add leeks, ginger and garlic.

Cook over low heat. Add stock. Simmer 10 minutes.

Add spinach. Bring to the boil. Serve hot.

Health Benefits Of Spinach:

Important for skin, hair and bone health. Provides protein, iron, calcium, magnesium and vitamin A. One of the best sources of dietary potassium.

Chicken Chowder

Serves; 6

3 tbsp unsalted butter

2 onions, finely diced

2 stalks celery, finely chopped

2 large carrots, peeled and diced

2 potatoes, peeled and diced

1/2 cooked chicken, shredded

2 bay leaves

1 sprig fresh thyme

freshly ground pepper, preferably white

1 1/2 cups fresh or frozen corn kernels

6 cups chicken stock or water

3 tbsp cornflour, mixed with a 5 tbsp milk

3 tbsp flat-leaf parsley, chopped

Method

Heat butter in a large saucepan. Add onions and fry until transparent, about 3 minutes. Add celery and carrots. Cook until softened. Add stock, bay leaves, thyme and pepper. Cook for 25 minutes on low heat. Add corn kernels and chicken. Add cornflour paste and stir in the rest of the milk. Add to soup. Cook 4 minutes. Adjust seasoning. Add parsley. Serve hot with French bread slices: grill both sides. Rub with garlic cloves. Brush with extra virgin olive oil and serve warm.

Health Benefits Of Sweet Corn:
High in fiber. Protects the body from cancer and heart disease.

Pasta Soup

Serves: 4

Ingredients

1 carrot, diced

2 potatoes, diced

1 stalk celery, diced

4 large tomatoes, peeled and diced

1.5 liters chicken stock

400g tin low salt tomato puree

1 cup dried cannellini beans (cooked for 1 1/2 hours. Drain.)
200g dried small tubular pasta
2 cloves garlic, chopped
1 small piece chili
fresh rosemary, sage, basil, finely chopped
freshly ground black pepper
1 homemade Italian sausage
extra virgin olive oil

Method

Heat 4 tbsp chicken stock with 2 tbsp olive oil. Add garlic and 'sweat' it for 2 minutes. Add tomatoes, potatoes, celery, carrot and stir well. Add remaining stock. Bring to boil. Simmer 20 minutes on low heat. Add cooked beans, pasta, chili, basil, rosemary and sage. Taste for seasoning. Cook a further 10 minutes. Pour into bowls. Drizzle with extra virgin olive oil and serve.

Health Benefits Of Pasta:
Contains selenium, a mineral that protects the body from cell damage. Contains manganese to metabolize carbohydrates and regulate blood sugar. Excellent source of vitamin B9, foliate.

Gazpacho Soup

Serves: 6-8

Ingredients

1 kg tomatoes, peeled, seeded, finely chopped

400g tin low salt tomato puree

500 ml homemade chicken stock

2-4 cloves garlic, peeled and crushed

3 tbsp white wine vinegar

1 1/2 tbsp. olive oil

red pepper flakes

fresh basil, marjoram, mint or parsley

Garnish:

1 large red capsicum

1 large green capsicum

6 slices bread, cut in cubes

1 small cucumber

1 large red onion

olive oil or rice bran oil for frying

Black pepper, freshly ground

Method

Place tomatoes in a soup tureen, or serving bowl. Add tomato puree, chicken stock, vinegar, olive oil and crushed garlic. Season with pepper and red pepper flakes to taste. Place in fridge.

For Garnish: chop cucumber, capsicums and onion into small cubes and place in individual bowls. Cover with plastic wrap and place in the fridge. Just before serving, heat olive oil in a frying pan and add bread. Fry until golden. Drain on kitchen paper. When cool place in a bowl.

Place the tureen on the table surrounded by the 4 bowls of garnishes. Serve soup and top with garnishes to taste.

Health Benefits Of Red Capsicum:
High in vitamin A and vitamin C. Helps the absorption of iron. Contains B6 and magnesium; decreases anxiety.

Celery Soup

Serves: 4-6

Ingredients

350g celery stalks, chopped

2 tbsp celery leaves

120g potatoes, peeled and cut in chunks

2 leeks, white part only, washed and sliced

25g unsalted butter

580 ml chicken stock

150 ml single cream

150 ml milk

black pepper

Method

Melt butter in a large saucepan over medium heat. Add celery, potatoes and leeks. Stir well. Cook for 10 minutes. Add stock. Bring to a simmer and reduce heat to low. Cover. Cook for 20-25 minutes. Cool. Place soup in a blender and puree. Return to pan and add milk and cream. Bring to boil on medium heat. Season with pepper. Heat though but take care not to boil.

Noah's Two Of Everything Soup

Ingredients

2 carrots, peeled, diced

2 parsnips, peeled, diced

2 onions, diced

2 cloves garlic, crushed

2 potatoes, diced

2 leeks, white part only, thinly sliced

2 celery stalks, cut thinly

2 bunches flat-leaf parsley, chopped

2 peas

2 beans

2 tbsp olive oil

Method

Heat a frying pan with oil. Fry onions and garlic for 3 minutes until tender. Add the rest of the vegetables. Cook over medium heat. Cook for 10 minutes. Add beef stock to cover the vegetables. Bring to boil. Reduce heat. Cover and simmer for 30 minutes. Remove from heat. Season with black pepper. You can serve this soup two ways. As is, with parsley to garnish. Or blend the soup with 1/2 cup light cream or 1/2 cup of milk to make a cream soup.

Soup Au Pistou

Ingredients

1 onion, chopped

3 tbsp olive oil

2 tomatoes, chopped

2 potatoes, peeled and diced

1.5 liters cold water

2 leeks, white part only, sliced

2 carrots, peeled and diced

1 cup cooked cannellini beans

250g green beans, cut into 5cm pieces

freshly ground black pepper

Ingredients For Pistou

3 cloves garlic, peeled

1 cup loosely packed basil leaves, washed

3 tbsp extra virgin olive oil (low acid)

Method

Prepare Pistou: Place oil in a food processor or blender. Add garlic and basil leaves. Blend to a paste. Place in a serving bowl and cover. .

Prepare Soup: Sauté onion in oil until transparent. Add tomato. Sauté for 5 minutes. Add water. Bring to a simmer on medium heat. Add potato, leek, carrots and cannellini beans. Simmer for 15 minutes on low heat. Add green beans. Simmer for 5 minutes. Season with freshly ground black pepper. Place in a serving bowl. Serve a teaspoon of Pistou on top of each bowl of soup.

Health Benefits Of Green Beans:

Contains vitamin K; helps promote proper blood clotting. Contains iron, which helps carry oxygen in the body and benefits immune function and energy metabolism.

Eve's Chicken Broth

Ingredients

1 small chicken

6 - 8 cups water

Pepper

1 onion

a few sprigs of thyme, marjoram or parsley

1 bay leaf

1 tsp lemon rind

1 tbsp uncooked rice

1 tbsp parsley, chopped

Method.

Wash chicken. Place in a large saucepan. Add water. Bring to a simmer. Add herbs and a whole onion. Bring to boil. Turn down heat. Simmer on low for 2 hours. During the last 20 minutes, add rice. Cook a further 20 minutes. Turn off heat. Cool. Strain. Flavor with pepper, lemon juice and add some chopped parsley.

Pumpkin And Coconut Soup

A rich Asian flavored soup

Serves: 4-6

Ingredients

500g (1lb) pumpkin, peeled and cut in cubes.

1 tbsp lime or lemon juice

1/2 cup hot water

1/2 cup onion, chopped

1 stalk lemon grass, finely chopped

2 cups thin coconut milk

1 cup thick coconut milk

1/2 cup fresh basil leaves

1 cup homemade chicken stock

Method

Place pumpkin in a bowl. Sprinkle with lime or lemon juice. Set aside. Place onions, lemon grass in food processor and blend to a paste. Place in saucepan with thin coconut milk. Bring to boil, reduce heat and simmer for 5 minutes. Add pumpkin and cook until soft and tender. Stir in thick coconut milk and basil leaves. Bring to boil. Thin the soup with chicken stock. Stir. Serve hot decorated with shredded basil leaves.

Health Benefits Of Coconut Milk:
Highly nutritious, rich in fiber, vitamins C, E, B1, B3, B5, B6, calcium and magnesium. Antibacterial compounds protect the body from infections and viruses.

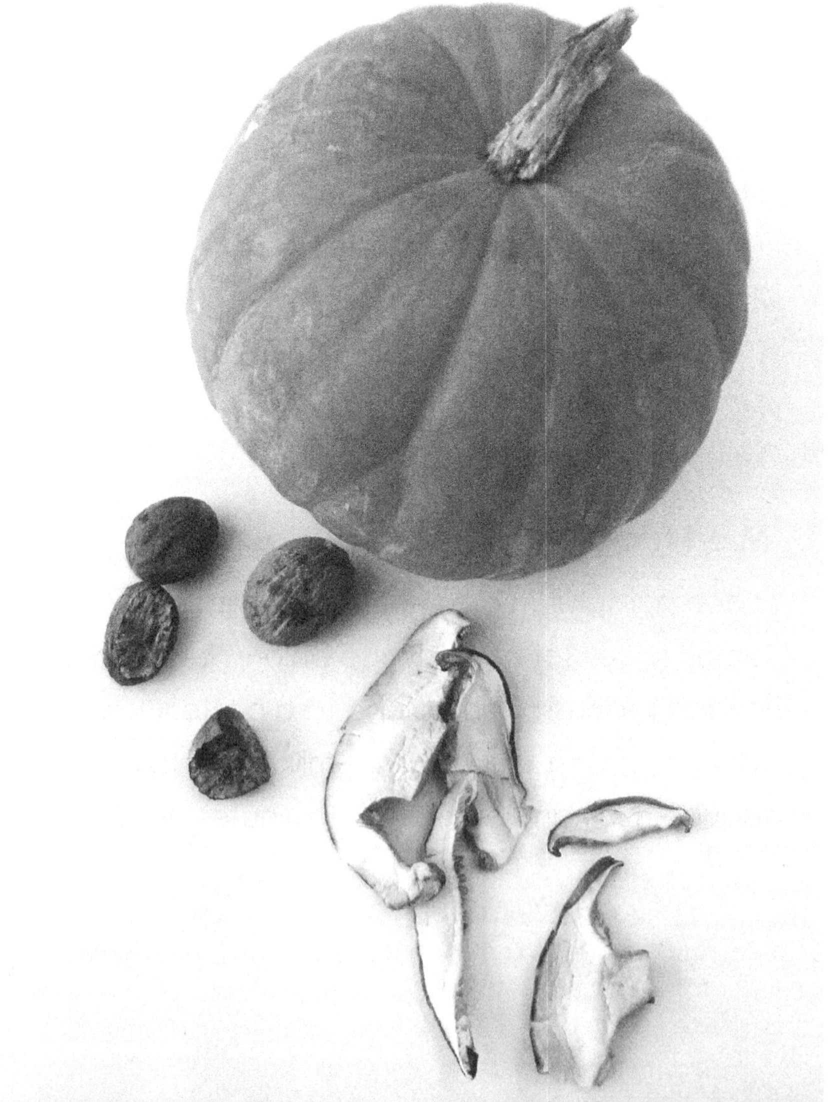

SALSAS VEGETABLES AND SALADS

Herbalicious Salad

Use magical fresh herbs and greens.

Ingredients

Any mixed lettuce leaves (radiccio, oak leaf, baby spinach) broken into small pieces
2 tsp mint leaves

1/2 tsp sage

2 tsp dill

2 tsp tarragon

1/2 tsp marjoram

1/2 tsp oregano

2 tsp chervil

30 ml red wine or balsamic vinegar

90 ml extra virgin olive oil

Method

Combine lettuce and herbs in a salad bowl.

Combine vinegar and oil in a screw top jar.

Use 1tbsp of herbs to 2 cups of lettuce leaves together with 15 ml (1tbsp) of dressing. Toss.

Health Benefits Of Lettuce:
Contains vitamin C, beta-carotene, omega 3, protein. Helps with insomnia. Alkaline forming; helps remove toxins and keeps acid/alkaline in balance for more energy, clearer thinking and restful sleep.

Avocado Dressing

Ingredients

3 tbsp lemon or lime juice

3 tbsp extra virgin olive oil

1/2 clove garlic

1 ripe avocado, peeled, mashed

2 tbsp white wine vinegar

freshly ground black pepper

Method

Combine all ingredients in a bowl. Pour over fresh leafy salad greens.

Health Benefits Of Avocado:
Contains 25 essential nutrients and is considered one of the healthiest food on the planet. Vitamin A, B, C, E, iron, magnesium and potassium help protect the body.

Slow Roasted Tomatoes

Good with grilled meats, bread, soups

Serves: 6

Ingredients

10 basil leaves

2 tbsp olive oil

6 tomatoes

freshly ground black pepper

Method

Shred basil leaves and place in the oil. Leave to marinate for 1 hour. Wash tomatoes. Place on a baking tray. Drizzle with basil oil, grind black pepper over.

Bake in the middle of the oven. 160C (320F) I hour. Cool. Store in a jar in the fridge.

Onion Jam

Makes: 1 jar

Ingredients

6 large red onions, peeled, cut in rings

2 tbsp olive oil

2 tbsp brown sugar

1/2 cup water

1 tbsp balsamic vinegar

1 cup dry white wine or chicken stock

2 bay leaves

2 cloves

1 clove garlic, crushed

freshly ground black pepper

Method

Heat oil in a frying pan. Add onions. Cook on medium heat until soft. Add sugar and 1/2 cup water. Cook 20 minutes until golden, stirring constantly to prevent onions catching on the bottom of pan. Add vinegar, stock or wine, bay leaves and cloves. Cook over low heat, stirring often. Cook 15 minutes until it looks like glossy jam.

Cool. Store covered in the fridge for up to 1 week.

Serve with grilled chicken, lamb, and beef.

Health Benefits Of Red onions:
Contains magnesium, potassium, manganese and vitamins C, K and B6. The outer layers of the skin contain concentrated vitamins, so peel as little of the outer layers as you can to get the most benefits.

Avocado Salsa

Serves: 4

Ingredients

3 tomatoes, seeded, diced

1 small red onion, finely chopped

1/3 cup coriander leaves, chopped

2 cloves garlic, crushed

3 tbsp light olive oil

freshly ground black pepper

2 ripe avocado, peeled

1 lime, juiced

Method

Mix tomatoes, onion, coriander leaves and garlic in a bowl. Season with freshly ground black pepper to taste. Mash avocados with a fork. Stir into the salsa. Add lime juice. Store and serve with toasted pita bread or unsalted corn chips.

Health Benefits Of Limes:
High in vitamin C, iron and minerals. Rich in flavonoids known for their antioxidant and antibiotic properties. Strengthens the immune system.

Orange Salad

Ingredients

1 bunch rocket leaves

1 red onion, sliced thinly in rounds

2 oranges, peeled, round slices, (save the juice)

3 tbsp pine nuts, pecans, or walnut pieces

Method

Lightly toasted nuts in a frying pan. Place rocket on

a serving plate. Place slices of oranges and onion on top of the rocket leaves. Sprinkle with toasted nuts. Drizzle with orange juice.

Health Benefits Of Oranges:
Contains vitamin C, vitamin A, potassium, calcium and vitamin B6. Boosts the immune system and reduces chronic inflammation.

Avocado And Citrus Salad

Serves: 6

Ingredients

2 avocados, peeled and sliced

2 oranges, peeled and sectioned

1 small bunch mint leaves

Poppy seed dressing:

1 lemon, juiced

4 tbsp olive oil

1 1/2 tbsp poppy seeds (make sure they are fresh)

Method

Cut avocado into chunks. Cut oranges into chunks. Arrange salad greens on a plate. Top with oranges and avocado. Combine poppy seed dressing ingredients together in a screw top jar. Shake well. Add a grind of black pepper. Shake. Pour over the salad and serve. Garnish with mint leaves.

Marinated Bean Salad

Serves: 4-6

Ingredients

2 cups cooked green beans

1 green capsicum, chopped

1 small red onion, grated

1 cup celery, sliced

Dressing:

1/2 tsp white pepper

3 tbsp sugar

6 tbsp white wine vinegar

12 tbsp extra virgin olive oil

1/4 cup water

Method

Combine vegetables in a bowl. Combine salad ingredients in a screw top jar. Shake well. Pour over the vegetables. Cover and refrigerate for 1 day.

Health Benefits Of White Wine Vinegar:
Protects against heart disease and cancer and may help slow the aging process. Vinegar acts as a substitute for salt in a low sodium diet.

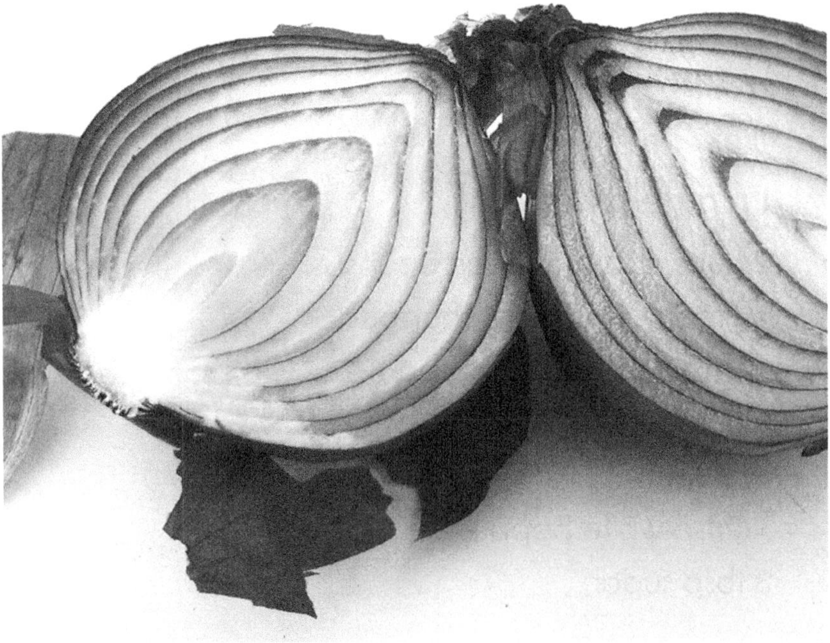

Mediterranean Vegetables

This is great with lamb and fish. If you have a big enough oven dish, it's easy to double this recipe for a crowd.

Serves: 4-6

Ingredients

400g fresh Italian tomatoes, chopped
3 medium red onions, peeled and quartered
2 red capsicum, deseeded, cut in thick strips
1 yellow capsicum, deseeded, cut in thick strips
8 small potatoes, skin on, parboiled 10 minutes
2 cloves garlic, chopped
big handful roughly chopped oregano
3 tbsp olive oil
freshly ground black pepper
fresh basil leaves, shredded

Method

Heat oven to 200 C. Toss vegetables except tomatoes in oil. Place in a baking tray and cook for

20 minutes. Remove from oven and add tomatoes. Toss. Return to oven and cook for a further 15 minutes. Remove from oven. Add freshly ground pepper and torn basil leaves.

Health Benefits Of Red Potatoes:
Packed with starch for concentrated energy. High in essential iron and vitamin C, zinc and copper for a healthy nervous system.

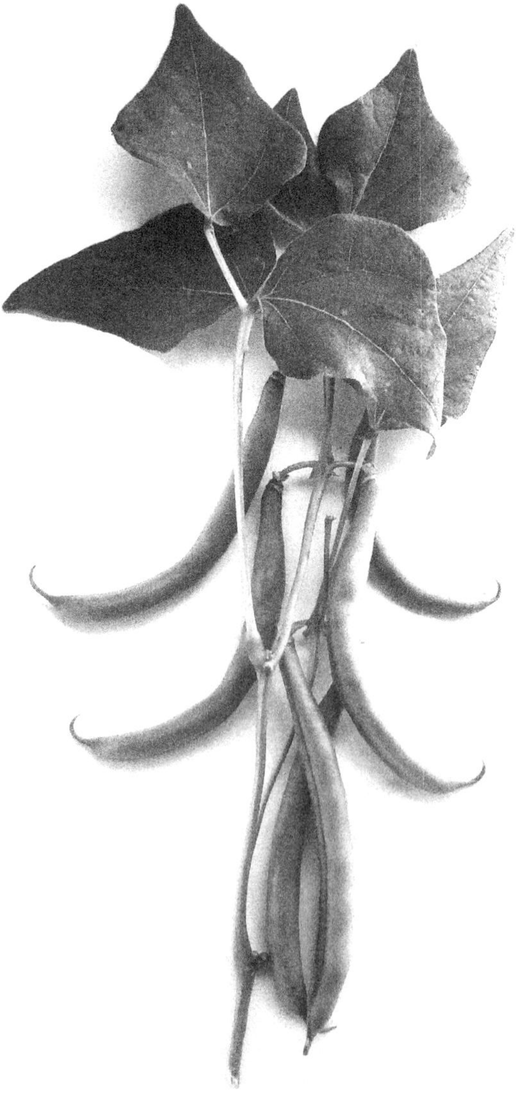

Tomato And Mint Salad

Ingredients

500g ripe acid-free Italian tomatoes, sliced

Juice 1 lemon

freshly ground black pepper

1/4 tsp caster sugar

Small bunch fresh mint leaves, washed

1/2 tsp grated lemon zest

cos lettuce leaves (or other variety)

Method

Marinate tomatoes in lemon juice, black pepper; caster sugar, lemon zest and shredded mint leaves for 30 minutes. Place two spoonfuls in a fresh cos lettuce leaf 'plate'. Serve on a platter as a salad or to accompany hot or cold meat.

Health Benefits Of Cos Lettuce:
Heart healthy with high levels of vitamin C and K. Contains potassium, fiber and folate.

Roasted Red Peppers

Ingredients

6 red or yellow capsicums

3 tbsp extra virgin olive oil

freshly ground black pepper

2 tbsp fresh basil, chopped

freshly ground black pepper

Method

Heat oven to 190 C. Place peppers in an oven dish and drizzle with a little olive oil. Place in the oven and grill until tender, turning until the skin is blackened and blistered. Remove from oven and seal in a plastic bag. Leave for 10 minutes. Place on a cutting board. Peel the skin off the peppers. Holding over a bowl to save the juice, cut the capsicums in half and remove the seeds. Discard seeds but keep the juice. Cut into long strips.
Mix remaining ingredients in a small bowl. Add capsicum juice. Arrange on a plate and spoon dressing over. Serve at room temperature.

Zucchini Fritters

Serves: 4

Ingredients

1 zucchini

1 large egg

3 tbsp plain flour

1/2 tsp baking powder

1 tbsp onion, finely chopped

1 clove garlic, crushed

1 tbsp fresh mint leaves, finely chopped

1 tsp lemon or lime juice

ground black pepper

1 tsp melted unsalted butter

extra unsalted butter for frying

Method

Grate zucchini. Squeeze juice out with your hands and discard. Place zucchini in a kitchen towel. Squeeze out any remaining juice (you can save juice and use in soup stocks).

Place egg and flour in a bowl. Mix until smooth. Add zucchini, onion, garlic, mint, lemon juice, melted butter and pepper. Mix well.

Melt butter in a heavy based frying pan. Spoon mixture into hot pan. Cook for 3 minutes each side until browned and cooked through. Serve with fresh tomato salsa. You can replace zucchini with sweetcorn (cut kernels from 3 fresh cobs) and use coriander leaves instead of mint.

Health Benefits Of Zucchini:
A good source of magnesium, fiber and folate.

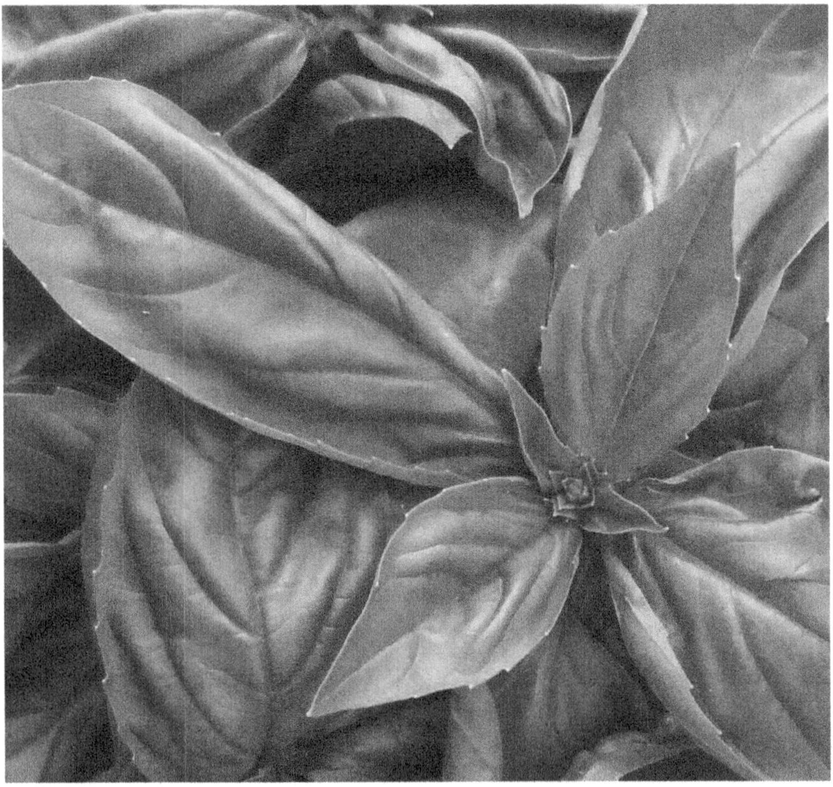

Spinach Tart

Makes 2 26-28 cm tarts

Ingredients

1 cup (250g) low salt cream cheese, or homemade ricotta, or mascarpone

6 eggs

1 cup milk

2 tbsp basil leaves

2 spring onions, pale part only, chopped

500g baby spinach leaves

1/4 tsp nutmeg, freshly grated

freshly ground black pepper

Ingredients For Pastry

2 cups flour

150g unsalted butter

About 4 tbsp cold water

Method

Heat oven to 200 C. Grease two 26-28 cm quiche or flan baking dishes.

Make Pastry: Place flour and butter in a food

processor. Process until fine breadcrumbs. Slowly drizzle in enough water to make pastry hold together in a soft ball. Take care not to over process or pastry will become tough. Roll or press pastry into the dishes. Blind bake, part cooking pastry until golden brown, about 10-12 minutes. Remove from oven and cool.

While pastry is baking, blend spinach, cream cheese, eggs, milk and basil leaves together. Add pepper and nutmeg to make a smooth green puree. Reduce oven to 180 C. Pour puree into pastry casings. Bake for 30 minutes until filling is set in the center. You can test this with a clean knife. Serve warm or hot. You can freeze the quiches.

To reheat from frozen, remove from freezer for 1 hour. Bake at 180 C for 15-20 minutes until heated through. Serve with tomato salsa.

Health Benefits Of Nutmeg:

Good for anxiety and depression. Fights fatigue and stress.

Bus Stop Potatoes

Serves: 4-6

Ingredients

16 small round potatoes, washed

1 tbsp extra virgin olive oil

1 tbsp fennel, cumin, or caraway seeds

1 tbsp fresh chopped rosemary or thyme

Method

Preheat oven to 250 C. Leave skins on potatoes. Place in a saucepan of water and bring to boil. Simmer for 10 minutes until not quite cooked. Drain. Transfer to a lightly greased baking tray. Squash each potato flat with a potato masher, so they look like they have been run over by a bus! Brush the top of each with oil and scatter cumin seeds, or caraway seeds and black pepper. Bake on top shelf of oven for 20-25 minutes until crisp and golden.

Irish Potato Cake

Ingredients

6 large potatoes

freshly ground black pepper

1 tsp thyme leaves

3 tbsp unsalted butter, melted

Method

Peel potatoes and cut in thin slices. Butter a 20cm flan ring and place on a buttered baking sheet. Arrange the potato slices in the ring in layers. Sprinkle with thyme and pepper between each layer. Pour melted butter over the top layer. Bake in a 190 C oven for 45 minutes or until golden brown. To serve, loosen the edges of the potato cake, by running a knife around the inside of the tin. Remove ring. Cut into sections and serve.

Health Benefits Of Unsalted Butter:
Rich in vitamin A (necessary for adrenal health). Great source of vitamins E, K and D. Protects against calcification of joints and hardening of the arteries. Provides a quick source of energy.

Hot Potato Wedges

These potato wedges are fluffy inside yet browned and crisp outside.

Serves: 6
Cooking time and preparation: 50 minutes

Ingredients

1 kg of potatoes, unpeeled, washed

1/4 cup (60ml) olive oil

Method

Heat oven to 200 C (180 C fan-bake)

Oil two oven trays. Cut potatoes into wedge shapes. Place in a large bowl. Add olive oil and toss. Place on single layers on baking trays. Brush with spice mixture of your choice. Roast uncovered, turning occasionally, for 30-40 minutes until crisp, lightly browned and cooked through.

SPICES FOR FLAVORING WEDGES

Lemon Pepper:

Combine 1 tbsp each of finely grated lemon rind and lemon juice and 1 tsp of black pepper.

Cajun Pepper:

Combine 1/2 tsp ground oregano, 2 tsp ground cumin, 1 tsp smoky paprika, 1 tsp ground turmeric and 1 tsp ground coriander powder with 1/2 tsp black pepper in a small bowl.

Garlic And Lime:

Place 1 1/2 tbsp oil, 5 garlic cloves (peeled and crushed) and 1 1/2 tbsp lime juice in a bowl. Whisk to combine. Add black pepper.

Bubble And Squeak

Ingredients

500g cold mashed or chopped, cooked potato.
500g chopped cooked vegetables (2 or 3 varieties)
1 cup diced cooked cold meat (chicken, pork, beef, or sausages)
60g unsalted butter
1 tsp white vinegar
freshly ground black pepper

Method

Combine potatoes, vegetables and meat. Heat butter in a heavy based frying pan. Add potato mix. Cook on medium high heat for 5 minutes, turning often. Flatten and smooth out mixture. Cook for a further 5-10 minutes or until golden and crisp on the bottom. Turn over. Cook for a further 5 minutes until the underside is golden brown. Sprinkle with vinegar and pepper. Garnish with fresh sage leaves which have been browned until crispy in a little unsalted butter.

Caramelized Onions

Ingredients

4 red onions cut into eighths

2 tbsp soft brown sugar

freshly ground black pepper

2 tbsp extra virgin olive oil

2 tbsp balsamic vinegar

Method

Heat oil in a frying pan on medium heat. Add onions. Fry on medium heat until transparent, taking care not to burn. Add brown sugar and stir until sugar caramelizes. Add balsamic vinegar. Stir for 5-10 minutes until the onions are glistening and syrupy. Serve warm or cold.

Roasted Beetroot Salad

Ingredients

2 beetroot, (beets)cut in 2 cm cubes

1 large red onion, peeled cut in thick rounds

6 cloves garlic, sliced

2 tbsp extra virgin olive oil

3 tbsp roasted pine nuts

1 cup rocket leaves

80g homemade mozzarella

Dressing:

100g frozen raspberries, thawed

1/4 cup orange juice

1/4 cup balsamic vinegar

Method

Heat oven to 190 C. Toss beets, onion, garlic and oil in a roasting pan. Season and bake for 45-50 minutes. Cool. Place in a bowl and toss with pine nuts, rocket leaves and dressing. Serve with mozzarella and extra rocket leaves to garnish.

Make Dressing:

Place raspberries, orange juice and vinegar in a small pan. Bring to boil over medium heat. Place in a blender and blend until smooth. Cool and strain.

Health Benefits Of Pine Nuts:
Rich in vitamin A. High in iron. Boosts energy levels.

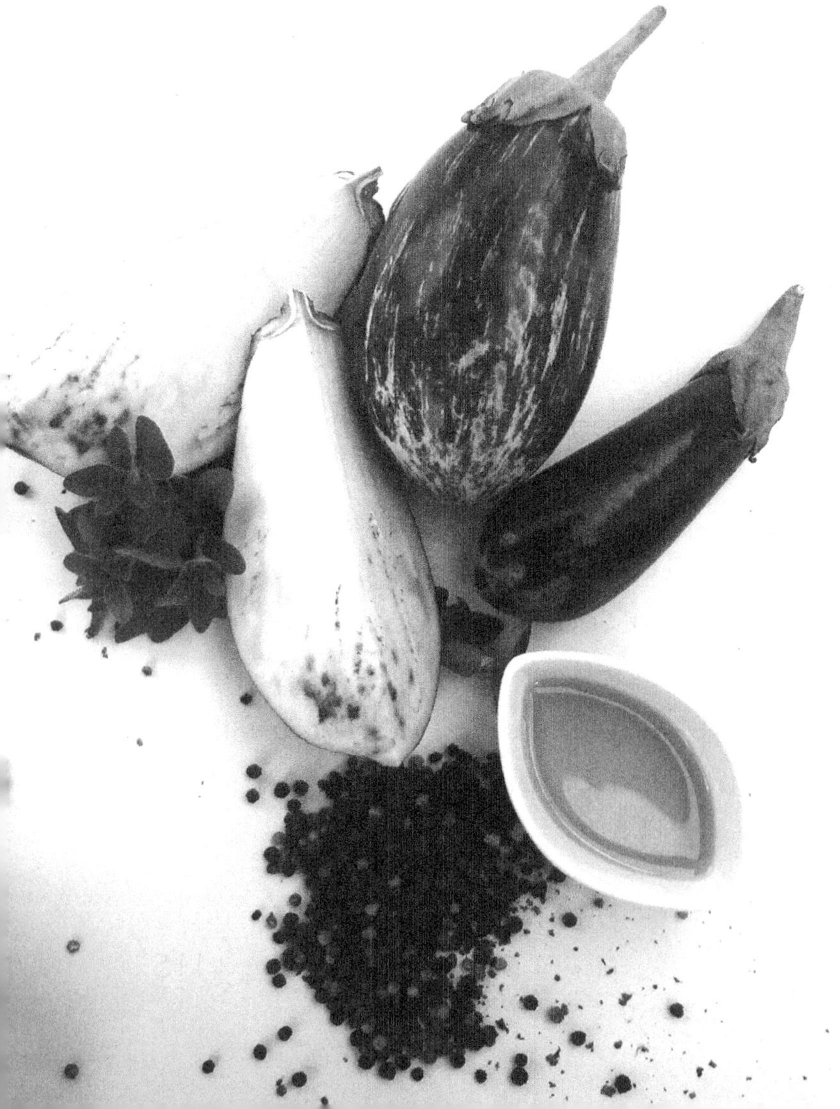

Beetroot And Orange Salad

Serves: 6

Ingredients

12 baby beetroot with leaves

1/2 cup balsamic vinegar

2 oranges, juiced

rind of two oranges cut in fine julienned strips

100g walnuts or pine nuts, roasted

2 tbsp finely chopped chives

Method

Cut leaves from beets. Wash and drain. Wash beets. Place on a baking tray with 2 cups of water. Cover with foil and bake at 190 C for 45 minutes or until tender. Drain. Cool slightly, then peel.

Cut warm beets into wedges and combine with balsamic and pepper to taste in a shallow heatproof bowl. Place in a turned off oven for 1 hour. Turn the oven on low to reheat the beets just before serving. Combine remaining ingredients, except walnuts and chives, in a saucepan and stir until warm. Tear larger beet leaves into pieces and arrange with small beet leaves on a serving plate. Top with beets and drizzle with warm dressing. Sprinkle with walnuts and chives. Serve.

Health Benefits Of Balsamic Vinegar:
Keeps blood glucose levels steady. Normalizes blood pressure.

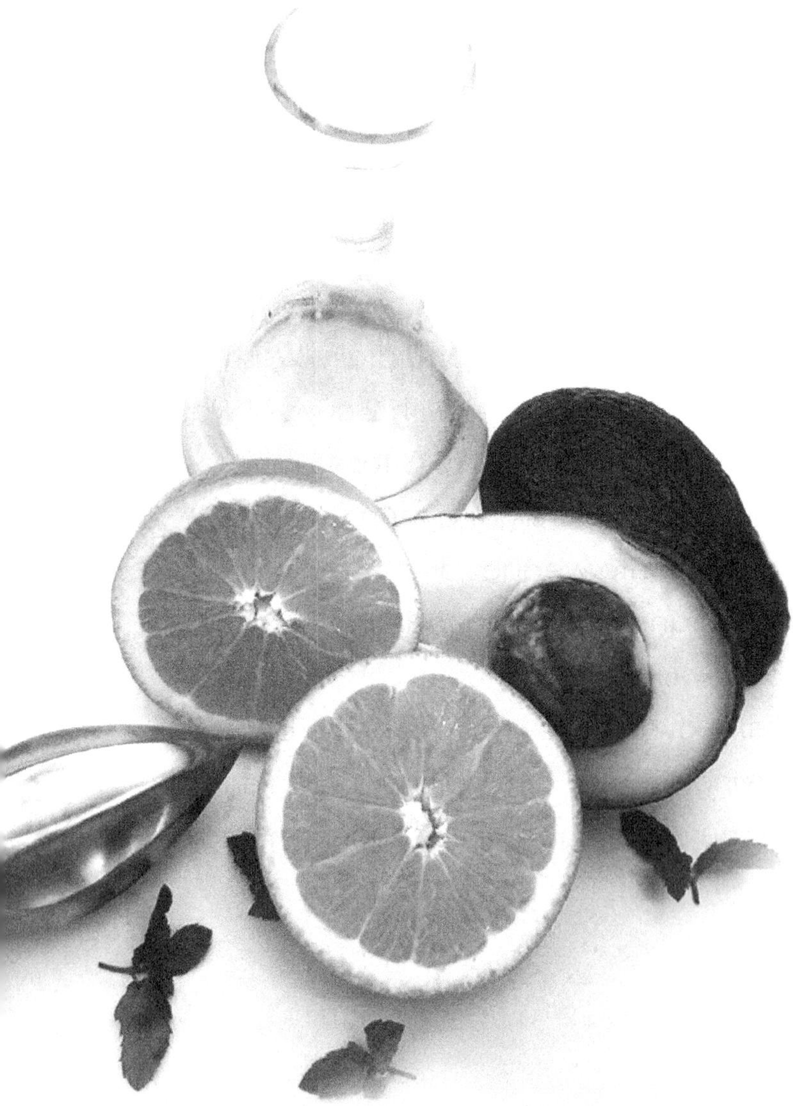

Best Potato Salad Ever

This is a bit of a family secret and comes from a hand written note to my sister, from a head chef in a local café she frequented in the 1960's.

Serves: 4-6

Ingredients

5 medium potatoes, peeled, diced

1 small red onion, finely diced

1 handful mint leaves, finely chopped

1 tbsp extra virgin olive oil

1 tsp white wine vinegar

1/4 cup toasted unsalted cashew nuts

Method

Cook potatoes until tender. Drain. Place in a bowl. Add mint, onion and freshly ground black pepper to taste. Add olive oil. Toss carefully. Add vinegar. Season to taste. Add more or less vinegar and oil to suit your palate. Chill in the fridge.

Pumpkin Salad

Ingredients

500g pumpkin, peeled and cut in 2 cm cubes

1/2 tsp cumin seeds

3 cloves garlic

freshly ground black pepper

2 tbsp extra virgin olive oil

1 bunch water cress, or mixed lettuce leaves

1 small red onion, thinly sliced

Lemon dressing:

1 tbsp lemon juice

2 tbsp extra virgin olive oil

1 tbsp honey, or fruit jam

freshly ground black pepper

Method

Heat oven to 190 C. Toss pumpkin, cumin, garlic, and pepper with 2 tbsp olive oil. Place in a roasting tray and cook for 20-30 minutes until pumpkin is cooked, but still firm. Combine dressing ingredients together in a screw top jar. Place onions and baby lettuce in a bowl. Add warm cooked pumpkin. Add dressing and toss ingredients until combined.

Roasted Eggplant Salad

Ingredients

1 eggplant, sliced
3 baby beetroot, cut in 4 pieces
1 red capsicum, cut in 4 pieces
1 yellow capsicum, cut in 4 pieces
1 yellow zucchini, sliced
1 green zucchini, sliced
1 red onion, cut in 4
fresh rosemary leaves
fresh sage leaves (or use basil, oregano)
1 clove garlic, crushed
extra virgin olive oil
1 tbsp balsamic vinegar
black pepper

Method

Mix garlic with olive oil and season with freshly ground black pepper.
Place vegetables in a large baking tray. Spread them out and brush with garlic oil. Place under a

medium hot grill. Grill until the skins begin to blister and darken. Remove from oven and toss balsamic through the vegetables. Place on a serving platter. Drizzle with a little olive oil and place fresh sprigs of herbs through the warm vegetables for garnish.

You can vary the vegetables and use whatever you have in your fridge: very thin slices of pumpkin, sweet potatoes, parsnips, carrots (cut lengthways), tomatoes cut in half, whole shallots, spring onions. Instead of grilling, you can bake the vegetables. Add rosemary and garlic to the oven tray. Then bake at 190 C for 20-30 minutes.

Health Benefits Eggplant:
Vitamin A, C, E and K, copper, iron, zinc, magnesium.

Lemon Garlic Mushrooms

Serves: 4-6

Ingredients

50g unsalted butter

2 cloves garlic, crushed

1 tsp fresh thyme

1 tbsp lemon juice

12 flat mushrooms, stalks removed

olive oil

Method

Place butter in a saucepan with garlic cloves and thyme. Heat on medium heat until butter melts and garlic is transparent. Take care not to brown. Remove from heat. Add lemon juice. Butter an oven dish. Place mushroom skin side up and brush with garlic butter. Grill for two minutes. Turn over. Brush with remainder of garlic butter until cooked. Serve on toasted bread or as a side dish to accompany red meat or chicken.

Mint Orzo Salad

Ingredients

200g orzo or pasta a riso (Italian rice type pasta)

1/4 cup raisins or currants

1/4 cup pine nuts

1/2 cup parsley, chopped

1/2 cup mint, chopped

1 red capsicum, diced

1/2 cup celery, chopped

Dressing

2 tbsp olive oil mustard

1 tbsp white wine vinegar

2 tbsp pomegranate molasses

2 tbsp orange juice

1/2 tsp curry powder

1/2 tsp ground cumin seeds

1 tsp whole grain mustard

Method

Place grain mustard, curry powder and cumin powder in a screw top jar. Add the rest of the dressing ingredients and mix well. Leave for 30 minutes for the raisins to plump. Cook orzo in boiling water for 7-10 minutes until al dente. Drain well. Place in a bowl. Add pine nuts, parsley, mint, capsicum and celery. Add salad dressing. Toss.

Spinach And Quinoa Salad

Serves: 6-8

Ingredients

1 tsp coriander seeds, toasted
1 cup white quinoa
3 cups cold water
2 large Italian style tomatoes, chopped
2 cups baby spinach leaves

For the dressing:

2 cloves crushed garlic
1/2 cup basil or mint, finely chopped
1 tbsp lemon juice
3 tbsp extra virgin olive oil

Method

Heat a frying pan over medium heat. Add quinoa and cook for 3 minutes until grains begin to pop. Remove from heat. Place in a sieve and rinse under cold water. Place in a saucepan with water. Bring to boil on medium heat. Reduce heat to low and simmer, covered until transparent, about 10-15 minutes. Drain. Make dressing in a screw top jar. Place quinoa in a bowl. Add tomatoes and spinach. Add dressing and toss.

Falafel

Chickpea patties. Serve with hummus.

Ingredients

450g chickpeas, soaked

1/2 onion

1 clove garlic

1 1/2 cups flat–leaf parsley, roughly chopped

1 cup coriander leaves, roughly chopped

1/2 cup mint leaves, roughly chopped

1/2 tsp freshly ground black pepper
1 tsp baking powder
2 tsp ground coriander seeds
3 tbsp ground cumin seeds
olive oil for frying

Method

Drain chickpeas in a colander. Run fresh water through them. Drain again.
Place in a food processor with onion, garlic, herbs, coriander, cumin and baking powder. Blend until the mixture looks green and holds together. Shape into 4 cm balls and flatten to form small patties. Heat oil in a shallow frying pan. Fry until crisp and golden on both sides, about 3-5 minutes. Drain on kitchen paper. Serve hot with hummus, tabbouleh salad, pita bread and a side dressing of tomato sauce (mixed with yogurt and crushed garlic).

Health Benefits Of Chickpeas:
Contain fiber, antioxidants, iron and protein.

Evergreen Café Hummus Salad

Serves: 6-8

Ingredients

2 cups chickpeas, soaked overnight

3 tbsp lemon juice

3 tbsp tahini (ground sesame) paste

2 cloves garlic, crushed

1/2 tsp cumin seeds, ground

2 tbsp, low-acid extra virgin olive oil

freshly ground black pepper

3 ripe tomatoes, chopped

1 cucumber, peeled and chopped

1 tbsp red wine vinegar

2 tbsp olive oil (for dressing)

1 tbsp flat leaf parsley, for garnish

Turkish bread or pita bread, to serve

Method

Drain soaked chickpeas. Place in saucepan. Bring to boil. Reduce heat and simmer until tender, about 30 minutes to 1 hour.

Drain peas and place in food processor or blender. Add lemon juice, tahini, oil, cumin, olive oil and pepper. Blend until smooth. Taste and adjust seasoning. Add more lemon juice, pepper or cumin to taste.
Place chopped tomatoes, cucumber, oil, vinegar and pepper in a bowl. Mix well.
Place hummus in a shallow serving dish. Spoon cucumber and tomatoes salad over the hummus. Serve at room temperature with bread for dipping.

Health Benefits Of Tahini:
Rich source of B vitamins to boost energy. Vitamin E and minerals, magnesium, zinc, iron and calcium.

Tabbouleh Salad

155g bulgur wheat

1/2 cup spring onion, finely diced

3 tbsp lemon juice

2 tbsp light virgin olive oil

1 cup flat-leaf parsley, chopped

2 tbsp mint, finely chopped

375g ripe tomatoes, peeled, finely diced

Method

Soak cracked wheat in cold water for 1 hour. Drain and squeeze all the water out. Combine with lemon juice, oil and pepper. Add spring onion, mint leaves and parsley. Season with pepper. Serve.

Health Benefits Of Bulgur Wheat:
Impressive amounts of manganese helps protect the body from free radicals.

PASTA AND RICE

Pepper Pesto With Linguine

Serves: 4-6

Ingredients

400g dried linguine pasta

3 red capsicums

2 cloves garlic, peeled

25g basil leaves

70g roasted hazelnuts

4 tbsp extra virgin olive oil

Method

Heat oven to 200 C.

Make pesto: place capsicum on an oven tray. Roast 20-25 minutes, until charred. Place in a plastic bag to sweat. Slip off the skins. Deseed. Place basil, nuts and garlic in a food processor. Pulse to a course paste. Slowly add oil. Add capsicum and process until smooth. Add extra oil if needed. Cook linguine according to the instructions on the packet. Drain. Toss in the red pepper pesto. Season to taste with black pepper and shredded basil leaves.

Fresh Tomato Pasta Sauce

Serves: 4-6

Ingredients

6-8 ripe Roma (acid free) Italian tomatoes
2 tbsp extra virgin olive oil
freshly ground black pepper
1 clove garlic, crushed, garlic,
bunch small fresh basil, washed, leaves only
spaghetti, 100g per person

Method

Heat water to boiling. Turn off heat. Carefully drop the tomatoes into the boiled water for 30 seconds. Lift tomatoes out. Peel skin. Cut tomatoes in half. Squeeze out the seeds. Discard. Chop tomatoes into small pieces. Place olive oil, pepper, garlic and tomatoes into a bowl. Add torn basil leaves. Leave for 1 hour in the fridge. Cook pasta according to the directions on the packet. Drain pasta. Place into serving bowls. Add tomato sauce and shredded basil leaves.

Basmati Pilaf

Serves: 4-6

Ingredients

1 tbsp extra virgin olive oil

3cm cinnamon stick

2 whole green cardamom pods

1/2 cup thinly sliced onions

1 cup basmati rice, rinsed and drained

1 1/2 cups water

Method

Heat oil in a medium saucepan over high heat. Add whole spices and cook, stirring until they make a popping sound. Add onion. Cook 2 minutes until translucent. Stir in rice and cook 1 minute, until fragrant.

Add water and bring to boil. Reduce heat to low. Cover pan tightly. Simmer about 15 minutes until water is absorbed. Remove pan from heat. Leave covered for 10-15 minutes. Fluff with a fork and serve with curries.

Spicy Couscous

Ingredients

25g unsalted butter
1 onion, diced
2 cloves garlic, crushed
1 tbsp ginger, finely chopped
1 tsp ground cumin seeds
1 tsp ground coriander seeds
1 tsp turmeric powder
1/2 tsp ground chili (optional)
1 cup nuts (almonds, pine nuts, walnuts)
1 cup dried currants (or raisins)
1 cup pumpkin seed kernels
fresh flat-leaf parsley

Method

Melt butter in a large frying pan. Sauté onion, garlic and ginger for 2 minutes on medium heat. Add spices and nuts. Cook for 1 minute. Add currants and seeds. Bring 1 1/2 cups of water to the boil. Remove from heat. Stir in couscous. Allow to swell for 2 minutes. Add chopped parsley and the spice fruit mixture. Stir well and serve.

Easy Couscous

This can be made in advance and re-heated in a bowl over boiling water, or in the microwave.

Serves: 4-6

Ingredients

2 cups couscous

2 cups homemade chicken stock (or water)

1 tbsp olive oil

1/2 cup raisins

zest of 1 lemon

2 tbsp mint, chopped

2 tbsp dill, chopped

1 tsp paprika

1/2 cup slivered almonds, roasted

Method

Place raisins in chicken stock. Bring to boil over medium heat. Mix the almonds, spices and lemon zest with the couscous. Put couscous into a deep bowl and pour in the raisin stock mixture. Mix well. Cover tightly and let cool, without uncovering.

When cool, mix in fresh herbs, fluffing with a fork to remove any lumps. Reheat when required.
Serve with grilled or roasted meat such as rack of lamb or roasted chicken.

Health Benefits Of Couscous:
High in selenium (protects the cells DNA from the mutating effects of toxins). High levels of potassium.

Potato Gratin With Garlic

Serves: 6-8

Ingredients

1 kg potatoes, peeled, sliced thinly

2 cloves garlic, crushed

3 cups milk

1/2 tsp nutmeg, grated

Method

Heat oven to 200 C. Butter a baking dish. Place

potatoes in layers. Season with pepper between layers. Mix garlic with milk in a bowl. Add nutmeg. Pour over potatoes. Dot with butter. Cover dish with foil. Bake for 45 minutes or until potatoes are cooked and the top is golden.

Health Benefits Of Milk:
A good protein and calcium source.

Potato Curry

Ingredients

4 tbsp oil

1 clove garlic

4 potatoes, peeled and diced

1/2 tsp sugar

1 tbsp coconut milk

1 cup water

400g can no salt tomatoes, liquid reserved

2 onions, sliced

1/2 tsp ground cumin seeds

1/2 tsp turmeric powder

1/2 tsp cinnamon

1/2 tsp cardamom

1/2 tsp black pepper

1/2 tsp ginger powder

Method

Fry onion in oil on medium heat until transparent. Add garlic and spices. Cook for 2 minutes. Add potatoes. Fry 2 minutes. Add tomatoes and bring to the boil. Simmer 20 minutes or until potato is cooked. Serve with rice.

Coconut Jasmine Rice

Ingredients

1 cup jasmine rice

1 cup coconut milk mixed with 1/2 cup water

2 lime leaves, chopped

1 small red chili, chopped

Method

The rule is for every cup of rice; use 1 1/2 cups of liquid. (You can vary the amount of coconut milk to water ratio to suit your taste). Cook rice in coconut and water according to the instructions on the packet (cooking time varies according to the rice you are using). Once the coconut rice is cooked, add spring onions and coriander. Stir with a fork. Then place lid on the saucepan and set aside for 10 minutes before serving.

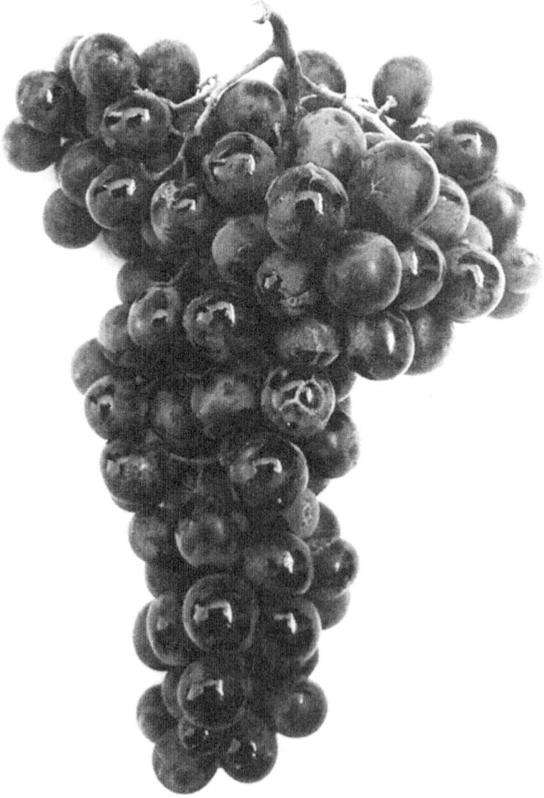

FISH

Fish In Grape Sauce

This dish can be made with any white fish.

Ingredients

6 fillets firm white fish

plain flour for dipping

1 large egg

30g unsalted butter

oil for cooking

1 tbsp shallots, peeled, finely chopped

1 cup seedless green grapes

1/2 cup white wine

1/2 cup thick style cream

white pepper to taste

Method

Place flour on a plate. Season with pepper. Dust fish lightly with flour. Beat egg. Dip fish into the egg. Heat oil in a frying pan. Quickly fry the fish until just cooked. Do not overcook.

Keep warm in the oven.

Heat butter in a saucepan on medium heat. Add shallots. Fry until golden. Add grapes. Add wine and cream. Increase heat. Cook stirring until the sauce reduces and is a thick, creamy consistency. Place fish on serving plates and spoon grape sauce over. Serve with mashed potatoes or rice.

Health Benefits Of Grapes:
High in potassium which helps regulate the body's fluid balance. High levels of vitamin C.

Noosa Beach Garlic Prawns

Ingredients

8 cloves garlic, finely chopped

1/2 cup light olive oil

24 raw prawns, peeled and deveined

1 cup white wine

2 tbsp lemon (or lime) juice

4 tbsp flat-leaf parsley, chopped

Method

Mix garlic with oil in a screw-top jar. Place in the fridge and marinate for 12 hours or overnight. Heat oven to 220 C. Place prawns flat in baking dish. Mix oil and garlic. Add wine and lemon juice. Cover with foil. Bake in oven for 5 minutes (or until prawns are pink and cooked). Sprinkle with fresh parsley. Serve hot with crusty bread.

Health Benefits Of Wine:
Contains high levels of antioxidants and potassium.

Fish Cakes

Soft centered and crunchy on the outside. Fish cakes can be easily made ahead of time.

Serves: 4-6

Ingredients

500g potatoes, cooked and mashed

650g cooked white fish, flaked

5 spring onions, finely chopped

2 tbsp flat-leaf parsley (or 2 tbsp basil)

finely grated lemon zest

1 egg yolk, beaten

1 tbsp lemon juice

For Coating:

1 egg yolk

140g plain flour

1 egg, beaten

120ml milk

100g dry breadcrumbs

3 tbsp olive oil

Method

Combine potato, fish, spring onions, herbs, lemon zest, juice and egg yolk. Season with pepper. Shape into 8 fish cakes. Whisk egg and milk in a bowl. Coat each fishcake lightly in flour. Then dip in egg. Then into breadcrumbs. Refrigerate for 30 minutes before frying. To cook, heat olive oil in a shallow frying pan over medium heat. Cook fish cakes 3-4 minutes each side until golden brown. Drain on paper towels. Serve with lemon wedges and salad.

More Fishy Ideas:

Spicy Prawn Cakes: Place 1 clove peeled garlic and 3 cm peeled fresh ginger in a food processor. Add 250g cubed fresh fish, 250g shelled raw prawns and 2 tbsp fresh coriander. Blend until just combined. Season with freshly ground black pepper. Shape into 12 prawn cakes. Chill for 30 minutes. Heat oven to 200 C. Cook prawn cakes on a greased baking sheet for 15 minutes until golden. Serve hot with lime wedges.

Fresh Fish With Lime Mayonnaise

Ingredients

2 tbsp plain flour

freshly ground black pepper

4-6 fillets boned, skinned white fish

1 egg

homemade toasted breadcrumbs

2 cloves garlic

2 tbsp lime juice

1 tsp lime zest

3/4 cup homemade crème fraiche

Method

Make breadcrumbs by placing slices of bread on a baking sheet. Bake in a 180 C oven until bread is dry and golden. Cool. Place in food processor and process to bread crumbs. Set aside. You can store any leftover crumbs in the freezer.

Prepare fish. Season flour with pepper. Coat the fish in seasoned flour. Mix egg and milk together. Dip floured fillets into egg mixture and then dip into breadcrumbs. Place in fridge until needed. Meanwhile make the lime mayonnaise.

To Make Lime Mayonnaise: puree garlic with lime juice, lime zest and crème fraiche. Add pepper to taste. Set aside. Heat oil and butter in a shallow frying. Fry fish for 2 minutes each side, or until cooked. Remove from heat. Place on a serving dish with lime mayonnaise, salad and oven baked potato wedges.

Zoe's Beer Batter For Fish

Ingredients

4-6 pieces fresh fish
250g plain flour
1 tsp sodium-free baking powder
1/2 cup beer
1 cup cold water
light olive oil, or rice bran oil for frying

Method

Place ingredients in a bowl and whisk to make a smooth batter.

Heat oil in a pan. Dip fish fillets in plain flour to coat lightly. Dip in batter. Fry fish until lightly golden on both sides. Drain on kitchen paper. Serve with lemon wedges.

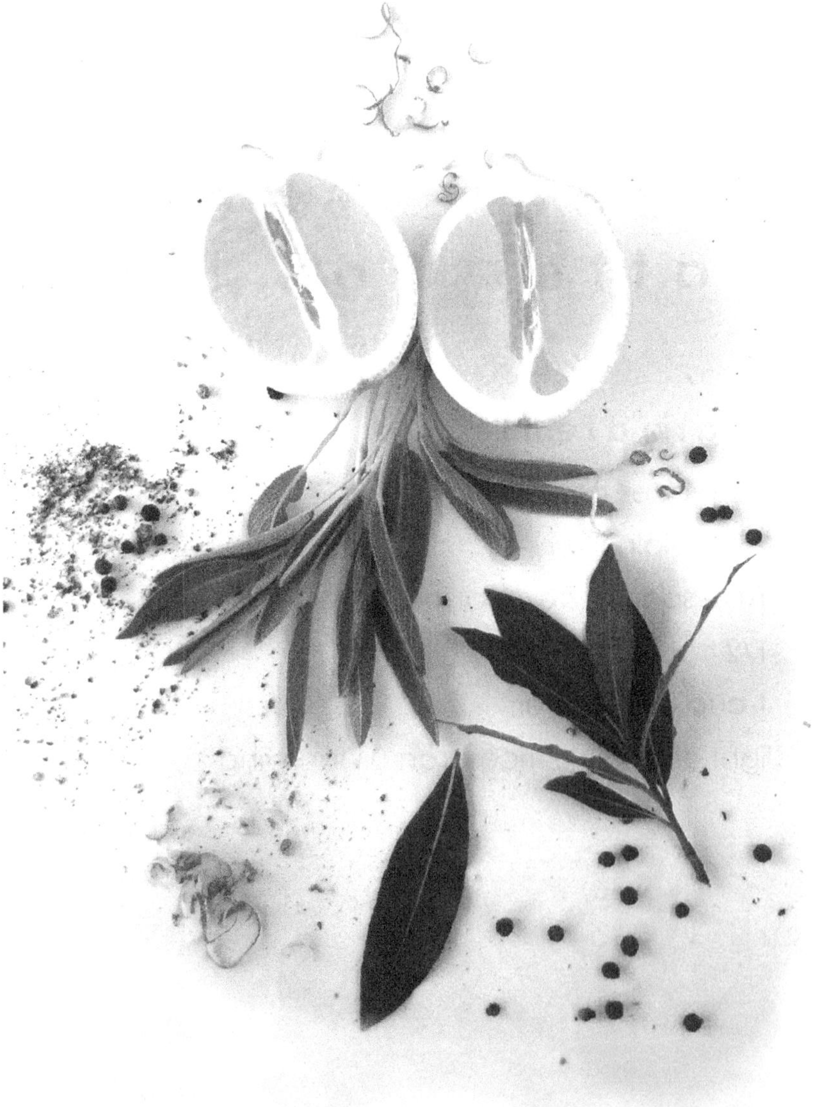

Palm Beach Prawn Salad

Serves: 4-6

Ingredients

12 green (raw) prawns tail on, peeled, deveined

1 lime (or lemon), juiced

4 tbsp coconut milk

1 tsp sugar (preferably palm sugar)

1 clove garlic, crushed

1 tsp fresh ginger, peeled and grated

freshly ground black pepper

2 tbsp fresh mint (or coriander leaves)

dried red chili flakes (optional)

Method

Heat a saucepan of water and bring to a simmer on low heat. Drop the prawns into the water. Cook until pink, about 2 minutes. Remove from heat and drain. Mix lime juice with 1 tbsp of strained prawn cooking water, coconut milk, sugar, garlic, ginger and pepper. Place prawns in a serving bowl, add dressing and toss through. Add shredded mint.

Poached Salmon Nicoise

Serves: 4-6

Ingredients

4 x 150g salmon fillets, boned and cooked

small handful fresh basil

small handful rocket leaves

3 large new potatoes, boiled, diced

4 eggs, soft boiled and cut in quarters

300g green beans, lightly cooked

freshly ground black pepper

24 cherry tomatoes, halved

Vinaigrette Dressing:

12 tbsp olive oil

6 tbsp white wine vinegar

black pepper

Method

Divide potatoes, beans and cherry tomatoes into 4 bowls. Season. Place dressing ingredients into a screw top jar. Shake well. Add a serve of dressing into each bowl. .

Tahitian Kokoda

Marinated raw fish in coconut cream.

Ingredients

600g fresh firm white fish

1 cup white wine vinegar

1/2 cup fresh lime or lemon juice

1 tbsp coriander leaves and stalks, chopped

1 fresh green chili, finely chopped

250 ml coconut cream

1 1/2 cups cherry tomatoes, halved

2 spring onions, thinly sliced

pepper

lime wedges for garnish

Method

Skin and bone the fish and cut into 2 cm cubes. Sprinkle fish with vinegar and marinade 1 hour. Rinse carefully with cold water. Drain on kitchen towels. Place fish in a bowl and pour lime juice over. Add coriander and chili. Mix together well. Set aside in the fridge for 15 minutes. Add coconut cream, tomatoes and spring onions. Mix and season with freshly ground black pepper. Place on a serving dish lined with crispy cos lettuce leaves. Garnish with lime wedges.

Health Benefits Of Cherry Tomatoes:

These are miniature versions of beefsteak tomatoes and equally nutritious. Vitamin B6, vitamin A. Contain lycopene to protect the body from cellular damage, osteoporosis and skin damage from UV light.

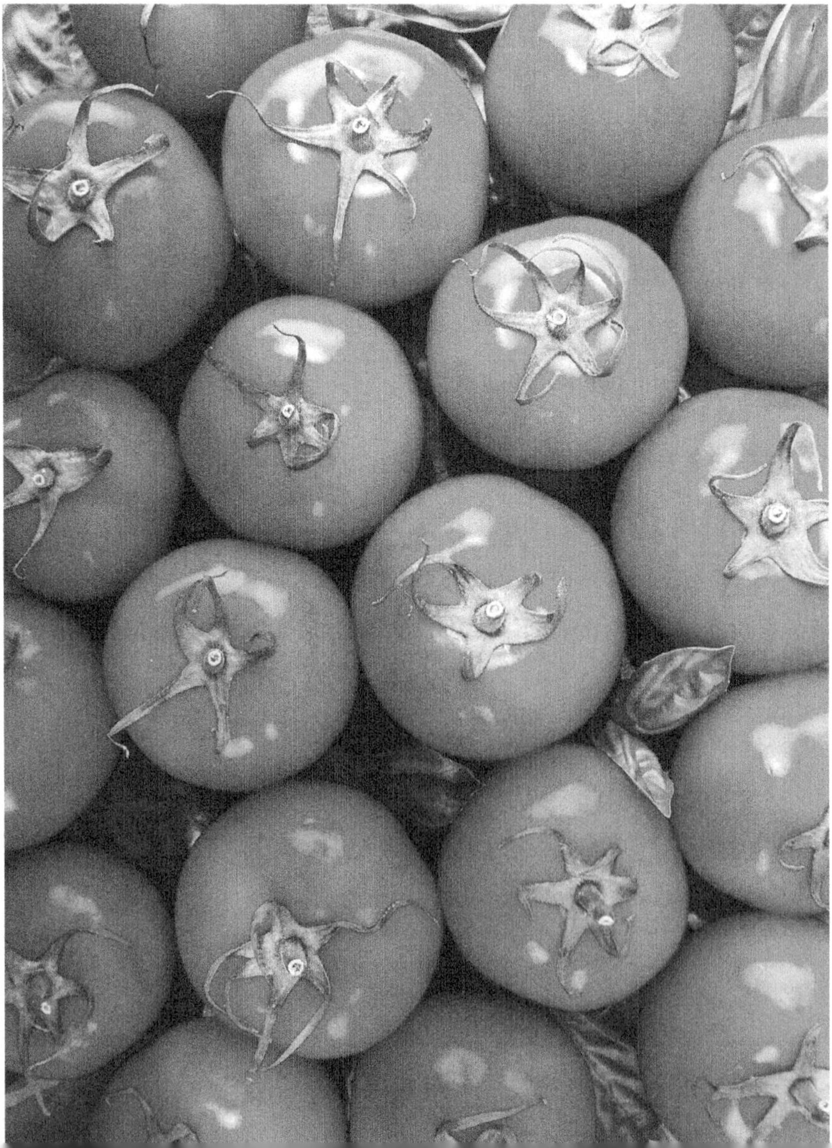

Moroccan Fish

Serves: 4-6

Ingredients

800g fresh fish fillets

1 clove garlic, crushed

1/3 cup coriander leaves, chopped

1 tsp paprika

juice of 1 lemon

1/2 cup olive oil

oil for cooking

Method

Dust fish fillets with freshly ground pepper. Place in a deep baking dish. Mix garlic, coriander, paprika, lemon juice and olive oil together. Pour over the fish fillets. Marinate in the fridge for 2 hours. Heat oil in a pan. Cook fish a few minutes on each side. Serve hot with lemon wedges. Serve with couscous.

Health Benefits Of Coriander:
Rich amounts of vitamins A, C and K. Thiamin, riboflavin, folic acid, calcium, iron, magnesium and potassium. Helps regulate insulin levels and can help relieve headaches.

Phu Quoc Island Prawn Cakes

Makes: 8 large or 16 small

Ingredients

700g fresh or thawed prawn meat

1 large egg or 2 small eggs

3 spring onions, chopped

2 small bunches of coriander

1 handful of mint

3 to 4 cups fresh white breadcrumbs

plain white (organic) flour

light olive oil , or bran oil for cooking

Method

Place prawns in a bowl. Add spring onions, coriander and mint. Cover and leave for 30 minutes in the fridge. Remove from fridge and add eggs and breadcrumbs. Shape into cakes. Coat in flour. Heat oil in a frying pan. Fry cakes in hot oil until cooked and golden. Drain on paper towels.

Cucumber Dip

Ingredients

1/2 stalk lemongrass

1 cucumber, peeled and chopped

1 small bunch of mint, finely chopped

1 small bunch coriander, finely chopped

1 small green chili (optional)

1 small red onion, chopped

2 tbsp sugar

2 tbsp hot water

2 tbsp lime juice

Method

Chop lemongrass stalk finely. Place with chopped cucumber, onion, chili and herbs. Mix sugar, hot water and lime juice in a small bowl. Pour over cucumber mixture. Serve with prawn cakes.

Health Benefits Of Prawns:
Low in saturated fat. Healthy omega-3 fatty acids help protect the body against heart disease.

More Fishy Ideas

Fish Burgers: Mince fresh tuna or white fish with fresh coriander leaves and a little grated ginger. Shape into burgers and grill on a barbecue or bake in a 190 C oven. Serve on grilled sourdough bread.

Marinated Fish: Take thick fillets of fish and marinate them in a little lime juice, some grated ginger, a shallot, finely chopped and 1 or 2 kaffir lime leaves, Steam fish in a bamboo steamer, fry or bake.

Baked Fish Fillets: Wrap fish in buttered tin foil or baking paper parcels and sprinkle with lemon or lime juice and any of the following spices.

Seasoning Ideas For Fish: Grated lemon zest, freshly ground black pepper, whole sprigs of herbs like dill, coriander, mint, spring onions, green peppercorns, flat-leaf parsley, grated fresh ginger, ground cumin, paprika, saffron, or Beau's blackened spices (recipe follows).

Beau's Blackened Spices

This is what Beau says about this recipe. "Whack em in a hot buttered frying pan with a hey ho. Turn them over and enjoy."

Ingredients

2 tbsp sweet paprika

2 tsp onion powder

2 tsp garlic powder

1 1/2 tsp white pepper

1 1/2 tsp black pepper

1 tsp thyme leaves, dried

1 tsp oregano leaves, dried

Method

Place in a hot buttered frying pan and turn them over, until aromatic. Cool and store in clean jars. Dip small pieces of fish or chicken (no more than 3 cm sized pieces) into the spices. Drizzle with a little olive oil. Grill, bake, barbecue or fry.

Salmon Orange Avocado Salad

Serves: 4-6

Ingredients

500g boneless salmon fillets

2 avocados

2 oranges

1 tsp orange zest, finely grated

1 red onion

salad greens

fresh coriander

Vinaigrette:

1 tbsp grated orange rind

1 clove garlic, crushed

4 tbsp olive oil

3 tbsp red wine vinegar

freshly ground black pepper

1 tsp cumin seeds, toasted

Method

Sear salmon fillets on both sides in a hot pan for a few minutes. Allow to rest. Peel avocados. Cut into slices lengthwise. Peel oranges. Cut into segments removing any white pith. Peel onion and cut in very thin rounds. Wash lettuce leaves and shake dry. Make the vinaigrette dressing by whisking the olive oil with orange zest, garlic, vinegar, pepper and cumin seeds together. Place salad in a bowl and toss with this dressing. Arrange in a bowl or individual plates. Place salmon, avocado, orange and onion on top. Pour over any remaining dressing. Add coriander leaves to garnish.

Health Benefits Of Cumin Seeds:
Contains B vitamins, iron and manganese.

Spicy Ocean Cod

Ingredients

cod or other fresh firm white fish (180g per person)

100 to150 ml extra virgin olive oil (mild, low acid)

1 1/2 lemons

1 tbsp lemon zest, finely grated

10 shallots, peeled and finely sliced
4 cloves garlic, crushed
1 tsp cumin seeds, toasted and ground
1/2 cup fresh coriander leaves, chopped
1/4 cup flat-leaf parsley, chopped
2 pinches freshly ground black pepper

Method

Combine all ingredients (except fish) in a food processor or blender to make a herb sauce.
Cut 6 squares of foil, large enough to hold the fish fillets. Place a piece of baking paper on top of the foil. Coat fish in herb sauce. Place on the baking paper. Spoon any remaining sauce over the fish. Wrap each portion into a parcel. Refrigerate for 4 hours. Take fish out 15 minutes before you bake it. Heat oven to 200 C.
Place parcels on a baking tray. Cook for 10-15 minutes (depending on the thickness of the fillets). Take care not to overcook. Remove from heat. Sit in a warm place for 3 minutes. Unwrap carefully. Spread tabbouleh salad on a plate. Place fish on top, including cooking juices. Serve with crusty bread or pita bread.

MEAT AND POULTRY

Pork With Prunes

Ingredients

1.5 kg pork, shoulder, cut in 4 cm pieces

1 bay leaf

1 sprig fresh sage

1/2 tsp ground black pepper

olive oil for cooking

2 medium brown onions, peeled, cut in chunks

1 1/2 tbsp fresh ginger, grated

2 cups homemade chicken stock

100g dried prunes, pitted or dried apricots

1 small bunch flat-leaf parsley

2 tsp orange zest

1 orange, juiced

Method

Heat oven to 180C. Grind black pepper over pork. Heat 1 tbsp of olive oil in a frying pan. Add pork and cook on medium heat for 5 minutes, or until browned. Remove pork and place in an ovenproof casserole. Add onion and ginger to the frying pan. Cook 5 minutes. Add stock, sage, orange zest and juice. Bring to boil and stir brownings on the bottom of the pan, to enrich the flavors. Add prunes or apricots on top of pork. Pour frying pan sauce over pork. Cover with a lid. Bake in a slow oven for 2 1/2 hours. Serve with potatoes and green vegetables.

Health Benefits of Prunes:
Rich in iron, and potassium

Pork And Veal Sausages

Ingredients

1 tbsp olive oil

1 large onion, finely chopped

2 cloves garlic, finely chopped

2 tsp ground fennel seeds

1 tsp ground coriander seeds

500 g minced (ground) veal

500g minced (ground) pork

1/2 cup breadcrumbs

1 egg

freshly ground black pepper

Method

Heat oil in a frying pan. Add onions and garlic and fry 5 minutes on medium heat until transparent. Take care not to brown. Add spices and cook for 2 minutes more. Cool.

Place onions and garlic in a large bowl. Add pork, veal, egg and breadcrumbs.Mix well. Season with pepper. Dust hands with plain flour. Dust a clean bench with flour. Break off pieces and shape into sausages. Leave in the fridge for 30 minutes to 1 hour. To cook, heat oil in a pan and fry, turning to cook until golden brown. Drain on kitchen paper. Serve hot with salsa or as part of a big breakfast with eggs, grilled tomatoes, grilled mushrooms, toast and homemade beans.

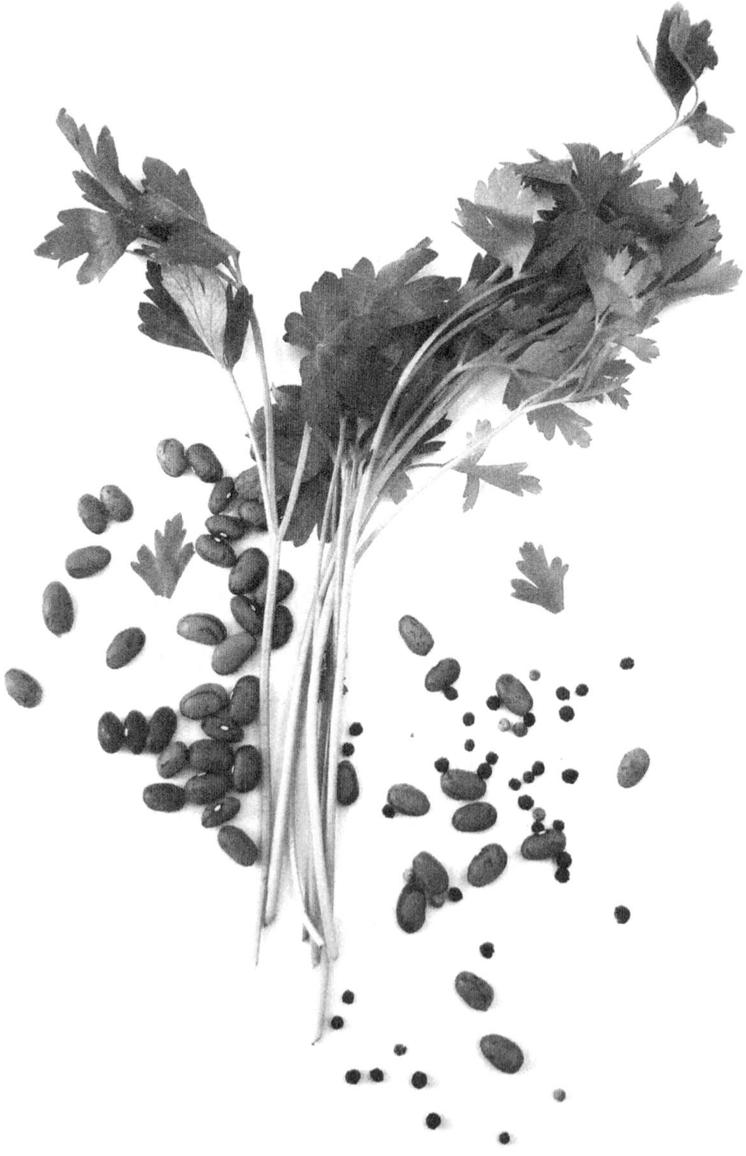

Beef In Beer

Serves: 4-6

Ingredients

1 kg chuck steak, cubed

1 tbsp olive oil

350g onions, peeled, quartered

1 tbsp plain flour

450 ml light beer

1 sprig fresh thyme

1 bay leaf

1 clove garlic

freshly ground black pepper

Method

Heat oven to 140 C. Heat oil in a pan. Add onions and garlic. Cook 3 minutes. Remove onions and garlic. Add meat to pan. Brown. Add onions and garlic back to pan. Add flour. Turn heat down. Mix flour with juices. Slowly add beer. Add thyme and bayleaf. Cover pan. Place in oven. Cook 2 1/2 hours without removing the lid to keep flavors in. The meat should be tender. Serve with potatoes.

Slow Cooked Beef Stew

Serves: 6

Ingredients

1.5 kg chuck or blade steak
2 tbsp plain flour
2 tsp sweet, smoky paprika
425g can tomatoes
2 onions, peeled and diced
2 cloves garlic, crushed
1 stick celery, finely diced
3 carrots, peeled, cut in chunks
3 potatoes, peeled, cut in chunks
1 cup beef stock or red wine
freshly ground black pepper

Method

Heat oven to 180 C. Mix paprika and flour together. Coat beef in flour. Place in a casserole dish. Crush tomatoes with a fork. Add to meat. Add the rest of the ingredients to the casserole dish. Cover. Cook for 1.5 hours. Check meat is tender.

Three Way Meat Stew

Serves: 4-6

Ingredients

1 kg chuck steak, cubed

1/3 cup organic plain flour

pepper to season

2-3 tbsp olive oil

1 onion, diced

1 garlic clove, crushed

4 cups homemade beef stock

125g button mushrooms, washed

Method

Coat meat in flour seasoned with pepper. Heat oil in a frying pan and brown meat. Remove from pan. Add a little more oil and cook onion and garlic in the same frying pan until transparent. Return meat to pan. Add 1 cup of beef stock to the pan, stirring and scraping the bits off the bottom. Stir until the gravy thickens. Place in a heavy bottomed saucepan. Add 2 cups beef

stock. Bring to boil. Reduce heat. Cook partially covered on simmer for about 1 hour.
Add mushrooms and reserved stock after 1 hour. When meat is falling apart and gravy is thick the stew is ready. Check seasonings. Serve stew as is, with potatoes or egg noodles.

To Make A Meat Pie

Use the stew recipe above to make a filling for this tasty meat pie.

Method

Heat oven to 200 C. Cool the stew and place in a deep pie pan. Add a sheet of puff pastry on the top. Bake for 20 minutes until pastry is golden brown. Serve with no salt tomato sauce or relish.

To Make A Potato Top Pie

Method

Cool the stew and place in a deep pie pan. Cook and mash 5 potatoes. Place mashed potatoes on the top of the stew. Bake for 20 minutes, until the top is golden.

Health Benefits Of Mushrooms:
Helps your immune system and nervous system. Contains vitamin C, D, B6 and B12.

Perfectly Easy Roast Beef

Ingredients

1.5 kg beef fillet

black pepper

(Optional: Rub 1 tbsp of balsamic vinegar and 1 tbsp of pomegranate molasses over the meat before roasting to create an extra savory glaze).

Method

Heat oven to 250C. Place beef in a roasting pan. Rub pepper over the beef. Cook in a hot oven for 20 minutes. Remove from heat. Allow to rest at room temperature for 30 minutes or up to 2 hours. Just before serving, heat through in the oven. Serve with salad and roasted potatoes.

Health Benefits Of Potatoes:
High source of potassium. Helpful if you are using drugs for Meniere's disease that reduce levels of potassium in the body.

Shepherd's Pie

Serves: 4-6

Ingredients

500g lamb or beef mince

1 large onion, finely chopped

2 stalks celery, finely chopped

2 carrots, finely chopped

1 tsp ground allspice

1 tbsp tomato paste

2 cups (500ml) beef stock

1 bay leaf

1 tbsp olive oil

freshly ground black pepper

1 kg potatoes, peeled, boiled and mashed

Method

Heat oven to 180C. Heat oil in a frying pan. Add meat and cook until brown. Cook onion, celery, carrot and allspice I minute. Add tomato paste, stock, bay leaf and pepper. Simmer 20 minutes. Place in baking dish. Top with mashed potato. Bake until golden brown.

Cajun Meatloaf

Serves: 8

Ingredients

1 tbsp extra virgin olive oil

2 onions, chopped

4 cloves garlic, finely chopped

1/3 cup no salt tomato paste

2 tbsp jalapenos, drained and minced

2 tbsp oven dried tomatoes, finely chopped

1 tsp cumin

500g lean minced (ground) beef

750g lean minced (ground) turkey

1/2 cup breadcrumbs

1/2 cup milk

Method

Heat oven to 180C.

Heat oil in a frying pan. Add onions and garlic. Cook 3 minutes. Place in a bowl. Add freshly ground black pepper, tomatoes, tomato paste, cumin and jalapenos. Add minced beef and minced turkey, breadcrumbs and milk. Mix well.

Grease a baking tin. Place meatloaf mixture in tin, smoothing the surface. Bake in oven for 1 1/2 hours until brown and crusty on the top. Remove from oven. Let sit for 10 minutes before serving with tomato salsa and salad with avocado dressing.

Sweet And Sour Lamb Casserole

Serves: 6

Ingredients

4 tbsp olive oil

2 onions, sliced

1.5 kg lamb shoulder, cubed

1 1/2 cups water

1/2 cup red wine vinegar

3 tbsp tomato paste

2 tbsp sugar

3 tbsp pine nuts

3 tbsp raisins

1 tsp freshly ground black pepper

Method

Heat oil in a frying pan. Add onions. Stir. Cook until transparent. Remove onions with slotted spoon. Set aside. Add lamb to oil and brown lamb well. Place onions and lamb into a heavy bottomed casserole dish, preferably cast iron. Deglaze frying pan with a little water. Stir to absorb juices. Add deglaze liquid to casserole. Add vinegar, tomato paste, sugar and remaining water. Cover. Simmer on low heat for 1 hour. Stir occasionally. Add pine nuts and raisins. Cook 30 minutes until the meat is tender. Skim off any fat. Season with pepper. Serve with mashed potatoes, couscous, or steamed rice.

Health Benefits Lamb:
B12 for nerve function, B3 for the nervous system and high protein for energy.

Marinated Butterflied Lamb

Ingredients

1.5 kg lamb leg, butterflied (bone removed)

Marinade

2 tsp ground cinnamon

1 tsp turmeric

2 tsp ground cumin

1/4 cup lemon juice

1 tsp ground nutmeg

2 tsp ground coriander

2 cloves garlic, chopped

1/2 cup olive oil

Lemon Dressing

2 tbsp mint leaves, chopped

2 tbsp coriander leaves, chopped

1 tbsp lemon zest

1/2 cup olive oil

freshly ground black pepper

Salad

A handful of baby spinach leaves

Eggplant, roasted, sliced

Method

Combine marinade ingredients and mix well. Place lamb in an oven dish. Pour marinade over lamb. Rub all over. Cover. Refrigerate overnight.

Heat oven to 200 C. Place lamb skin side up in a roasting pan. Use the same marinade for basting. Spoon marinade over. Roast the lamb for 200 C for 35-40 minutes or until cooked. Remove. Let the meat rest for 10 minutes before slicing.

Make a salad of leafy greens and roasted eggplant. Place dressing ingredients in a screw top jar. Toss though salad. Serve lamb with lemon dressed salad and couscous.

Jean's French Country Chicken Stew

Serves: 4-6

Ingredients

free range chicken (5 drumsticks, 5 thighs)

plain white flour

1 tbsp olive oil

1 tbsp butter

2 leeks, white part only, sliced

2 large carrot, chopped

4 stalks celery, chopped

1 1/2 cup chicken broth

400g tinned Italian style tomatoes

4 medium potatoes, diced

4 sprigs fresh thyme

4 sprigs flat-leaf parsley

freshly ground black pepper

Method

Wash chicken pieces and pat dry. Lightly dust with flour. In a large casserole, melt butter and oil together on medium heat on the cook-top. Add chicken pieces and brown. Remove from pan. Add leeks and cook on low heat for 10 minutes. Add carrots and celery. Cook 10 minutes. Add stock and let the stock come to the boil. Cook for 2 minutes. Add tomatoes, herbs and potatoes. Heat through. Add chicken pieces back to the casserole. Cover with a tight fitting lid. Simmer over low heat for 1 hour. Add thyme. Cook a further 1/2 hour, or until cooked.

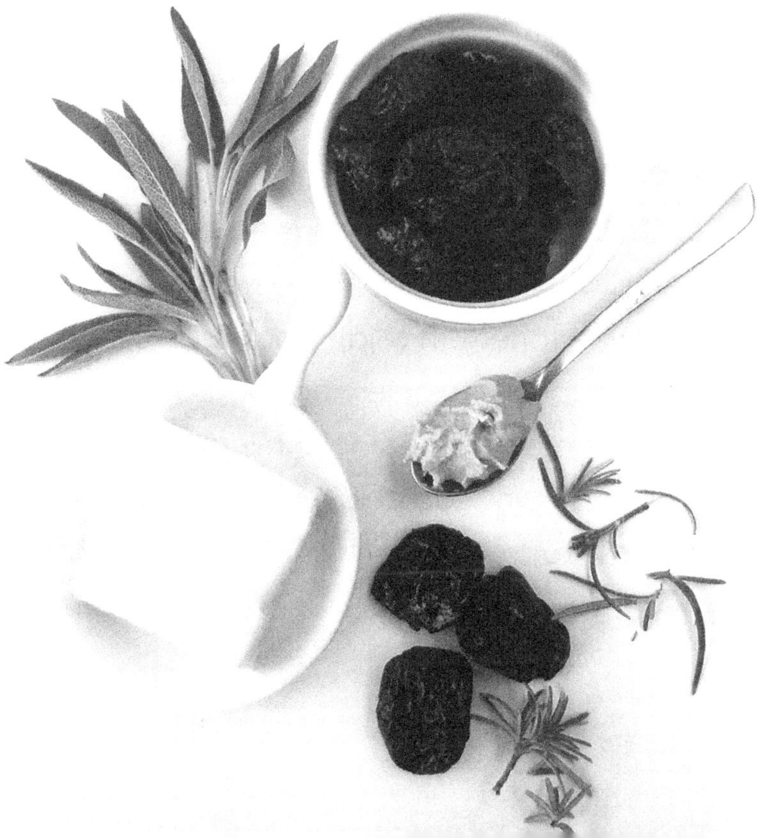

40 Garlic Roast Chicken

Serves: 4-6

Ingredients

1 large organic/free-range chicken

1 bay leaf

3 tbsp extra virgin olive oil

40 whole cloves garlic (3 heads) unpeeled

Thyme, rosemary, sage and/or parsley sprigs

2 red capsicums, deseeded, chopped roughly

2 celery stalks, roughly chopped

freshly ground black pepper

1 1/2 cups homemade chicken stock

Method

Wash and dry chicken. Place 2 bay leaves inside the cavity. Heat olive oil in a large oven-proof casserole (one with a lid). Add garlic cloves, herbs, capsicums, celery and season with pepper. Cook on medium heat for 5 minutes taking care to brown. Add chicken stock and bring to the boil. Reduce heat to low and simmer for 5 minutes. Remove from heat and place chicken in the casserole, breast side up. Spoon herb and vegetable juice over the chicken to coat. Cover with a tight fitting lid and seal with kitchen foil to keep the juices in.

Bake in a 180C oven for 1 hour or until chicken is cooked. Remove chicken to a serving plate. Spoon vegetables around and spoon cooking juices over. Serve with crusty bread to dip in the juices.

Health Benefits Of Garlic:

Garlic contains photochemical compounds which are thought to help eliminate potential cancerous substances from the body. Garlic has a long history of curative effects.

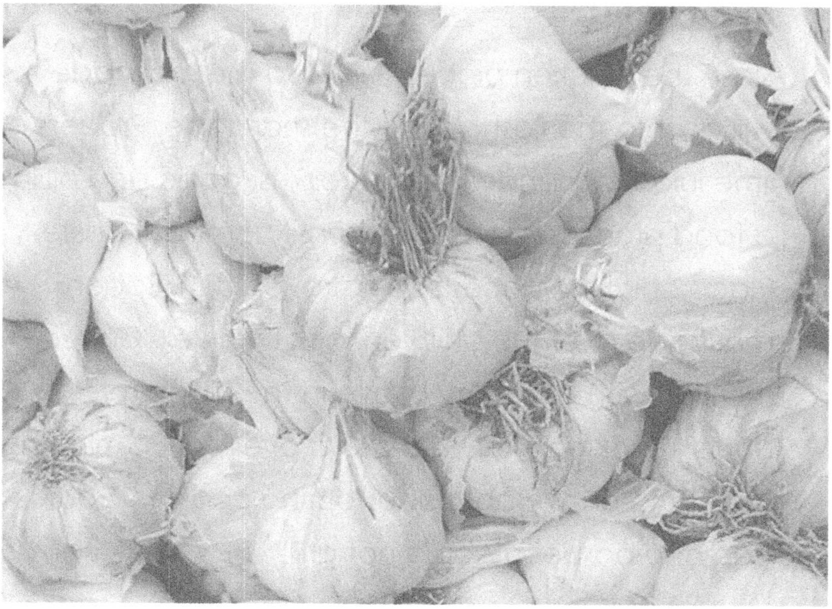

Lime Marinated Chicken

Ingredients

1 kg chicken pieces

2 cups coriander roughly chopped

2 tsp whole black pepper corns

3 cloves garlic, peeled

5 tbsp lime juice

1 tsp grated lime zest

60 ml olive oil

Method

Slash the chicken pieces a little so the marinade will go into the flesh. Make the marinade. Process lime juice, coriander, peppercorns, garlic and oil in a food processor or blender until a smooth paste. Place chicken pieces in a flat oven dish. Spoon marinade over the chicken, coating well. Cover the dish with cling film. Leave in the fridge for 3 hours. Cook chicken in a 220 C oven for 30 minutes, turning to brown both sides during cooking. You can also barbecue on a hot grill.

Chicken And Peach Salad

Serves: 4-6

Ingredients

1 roasted organic chicken

2 cos lettuces, torn into pieces

3 fresh peaches or 6 fresh apricots, cut in slices

2 spring onions (white part only), finely chopped

1/2 cup unsalted pistachio nuts, or walnuts

1/4 cup coriander leaves, roughly chopped

1/4 cup mint leaves, finely chopped

Orange dressing:

2 tsp cumin seeds, toasted

1 tsp fresh ginger, grated

2 lemons, juiced

1 tsp lemon zest

4 tbsp extra virgin olive oil

ground black pepper

Method

Make orange dressing. Place ingredients in a screw top jar and shake. Set aside.

Prepare chicken. Remove meat from chicken and save bones and skin to make chicken stock. Discard fat. Shred chicken into bite-size pieces. Place in a serving bowl. Add dressing and toss. Add chicken. Place cos lettuce on a serving platter. Spoon chicken on top. Serve.

Health Benefits Peaches:
Contains vitamin C, A and fiber.

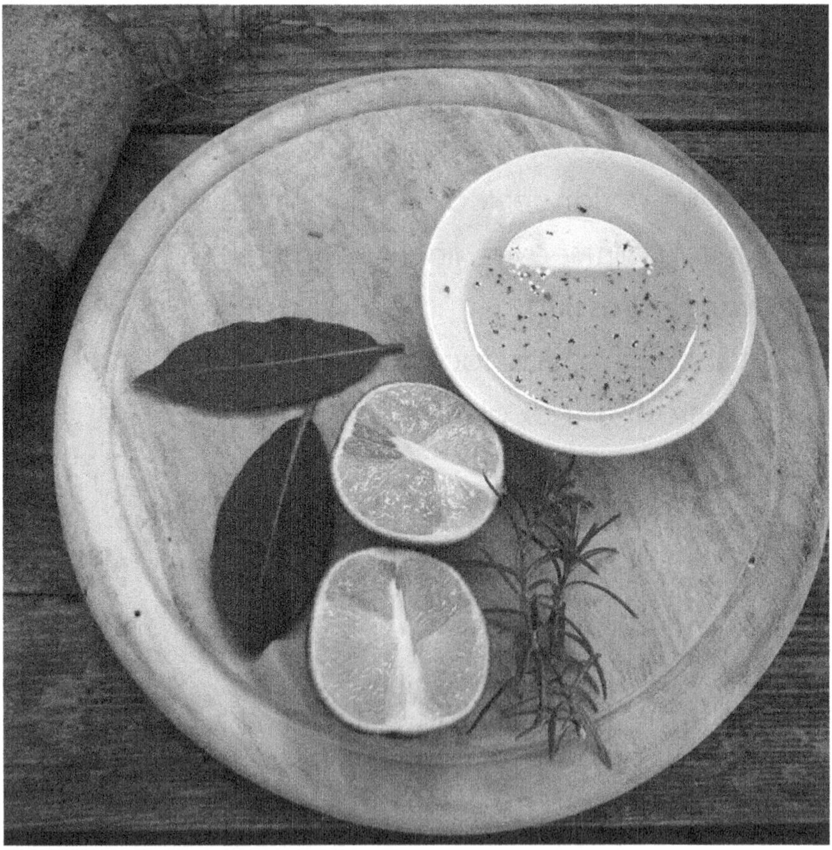

Baked Honey Lemon Chicken

Ingredients

16 free-range chicken wings (tips removed)

125 ml lemon juice

6 cloves garlic, crushed

1/4 cup honey

Method

Heat oven to 200 C. Place wings in an oven baking dish. Roast for 30 minutes. Place garlic, lemon, honey in a bowl. Stir until honey is melted. Pour over wings and coat well. Return to oven and bake for 15 minutes until brown and cooked. Add a grind of black pepper. Serve with salad.

Hanoi Chicken Noodle Salad

Serves: 6

Ingredients

For The Chicken:

6 chicken breasts, cut in half lengthwise

5 cloves garlic, peeled, finely chopped

1 cup coconut cream

5 tbsp lime juice (or lemon)

1 tsp ground turmeric

1 tbsp palm sugar, grated

2 tbsp coriander stalks, chopped

1 cup long-strand desiccated coconut

Method

Mix all together and coat chicken. Heat oven to 200 C. Lightly oil a baking tray. Place chicken on tray. Bake for 20 minutes.

Prepare Noodles:

350g flat Chinese egg noodles, cooked al dente and drained.

Toss Noodles With The Following Ingredients:

4 tsp sesame oil

2 sticks celery, thinly sliced

150g snow peas

5 spring onions, finely sliced

20 basil leaves, torn

1 tbsp Vietnamese mint

150 ml rice vinegar

4 cloves garlic. Finely chopped

4 tbsp palm sugar, grated

1/2 cup cashews, roasted for garnish

Basil and Vietnamese mint for garnish

To serve:

Place noodles on a serving plate. Place hot chicken on top. Garnish with nuts and herb leaves. Serve warm or chilled.

Sophie's Chicken In A Pot

Ingredients

1 free-range chicken

2 slices bread

1/2 cup milk

1 homemade no-salt spicy sausage

2 tbsp flat-leaf parsley

1 egg

1/2 tsp nutmeg, freshly grated

250g minced pork (chicken or veal)

6 carrots, peeled, cut in chunks

2 parsnips, peeled, cut in chunks

3 stalks celery, roughly chopped

2 leeks, while part only, sliced

2 small onions, cut in chunks

6 small potatoes, cut in chunks

sprigs of fresh herbs (marjoram, rosemary)

freshly ground black pepper

Method

Soak bread in milk. Squeeze dry.

Beat bread, egg, parsley, crumbled sausage, nutmeg, herbs sprigs and minced pork (or minced chicken, or veal) together. Wash and dry the chicken. Using the handle of a wooden spoon, carefully loosen the skin covering the breast to make a pocket for the stuffing. Stuff the bread mixture carefully between the skin and the breast. Place chicken in a large casserole with vegetables. Season with pepper. Add enough boiling water just to cover the chicken.

Bring to boil. Skim surface. Reduce heat. Simmer covered for 1 1/2 hours on low heat or until chicken is cooked. Remove from heat.

Carve in generous portions. Place vegetables on a serving dish. Place chicken pieces on top. Spoon stock over. Garnish with ground black pepper and fresh herb leaves. Serve this French country stew with crusty bread.

Roast Chicken Salad

Serves: 4-6

Ingredients

1.5 kg free range chicken

4 cloves garlic, crushed

1 sprig fresh thyme

1/2 lemon

4 tbsp olive oil

black pepper

Method

Heat oven to 200 C. Wash and dry chicken. Place lemon, thyme and garlic inside the chicken. Grind black pepper over chicken. Rub olive oil over chicken. Place chicken in roasting pan breast side down. Pour 1 cup of water over chicken. Roast 30 minutes. Turn chicken over. Roast a further 30 minutes. Baste often. Remove from oven. Take out lemon and herbs and discard. Skim fat from pan. Save meat juices. Set aside. Prepare dressing.

Roast Tomato Dressing

1/2 cup olive oil
Juice of 1/2 lemon
1/2 tsp sweet paprika
1 clove garlic, finely chopped
4 tomatoes

Method

Roast tomatoes at 200 C in a little olive oil until the collapse. Remove seeds. Place in a blender or food processor with paprika, garlic, olive oil and lemon juice. Puree until smooth. Add a pinch of sugar to taste and pepper.

Salad

Salad greens with your choice of ingredients. Roasted capsicums, or artichoke hearts; chopped cucumber, tomato and/or red onion. Fresh herbs: parsley, basil and/or mint leaves.

Place the salad ingredients together on a large platter. Cut chicken into large pieces and arrange on salad. Pour juices from roasting pan over chicken. Drizzle tomato dressing over.

Saigon Steamed Lemongrass Chicken

Serves: 4-6

Ingredients

8 boneless, skinless chicken thighs

2 tbsp coriander root, finely chopped

1 clove garlic

3 cm fresh ginger, peeled, cut in strips

1 lemongrass stalk, thinly sliced on diagonal

1 tbsp spring onion, finely chopped

12 fresh broccoli florets

lime halves, to garnish

Sesame Dressing

1 tbsp olive oil

2 tbsp lime juice

1 tbsp coriander leaves, finely chopped

1 tbsp sesame seeds, toasted in pan till golden

ground black pepper

Method

Fill a saucepan with water until the water level is 5cm. Bring to boil. Place chicken in a lightly greased steamer or bamboo steamer basket. Sprinkle coriander root, garlic, ginger, lemongrass and onion over the chicken. Place lid on steamer. Steam chicken for 30-40 minutes taking care not to overcook. Keep checking the water so it doesn't boil dry. When chicken is almost cooked add broccoli (or your choice of other vegetables). Replace lid and steam for a further 10 minutes. To make dressing combine ingredients, taste and adjust seasoning. Arrange chicken and greens on a serving plate. Pour dressing over steamed chicken. Serve with lime halves and coconut steamed rice.

Health Benefits Of Broccoli:
High levels of vitamin K and A.

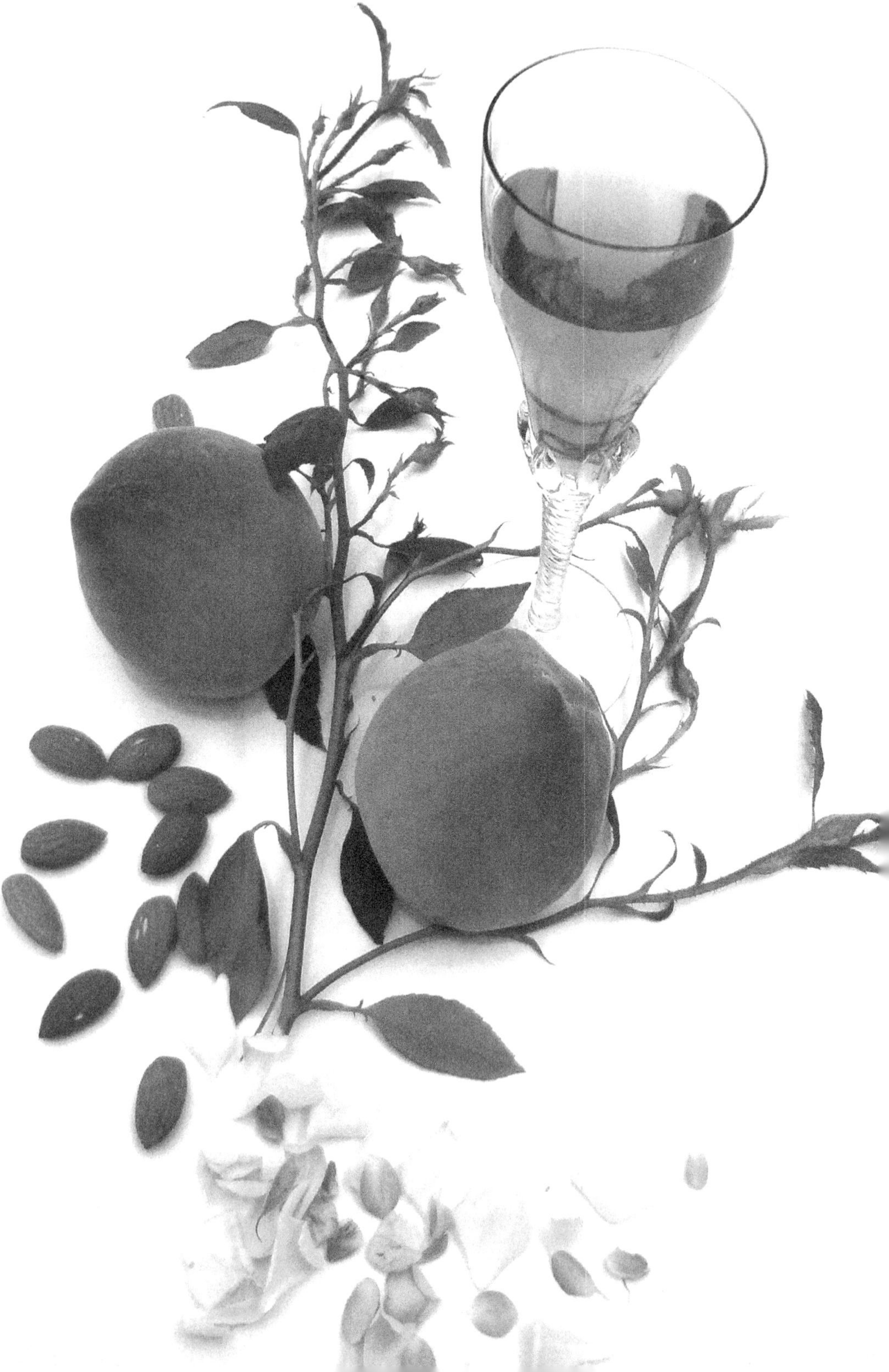

SWEET THINGS

Sydney Fruit Salad

Ingredients

rind of 1 lemon, cut in thin strips

2 cups water

400 ml orange or apple juice

2 tbsp sugar

1 vanilla bean, split in half lengthwise

1 tbsp fresh ginger, grated

2 stalks lemon grass

5 passion fruit

Selected fruit in season: Pineapple, mango, peach, strawberries, berries, kiwi fruit, banana, grapes
Extra mint leaves

Method

Put water, juice, sugar, ginger, vanilla, lemon rind, and lemongrass in a saucepan. Bring to the boil. Simmer 15 minutes. Cool. Cover and refrigerate to chill, preferably overnight.

Place passionfruit in sieve. Discard pulp and seeds. Add passionfruit juice to the chilled syrup.

Cut fruit into pieces. Place in a serving bowl. Spoon lemongrass and passionfruit syrup over the fruit.

Health Benefits Of Passionfruit:
Good source of dietary fiber, vitamin C, vitamin A and rich in potassium.

Lemon Pudding

Delicious citrus self-saucing pudding.

Serves: 4-6

Ingredients

1 tbsp unsalted butter

1/2 cup sugar

2 tbsp plain flour

juice of two lemons (or limes)

grated rind of 1 lemon (or lime)

1 cup milk

2 large eggs (separated)

Method

Beat eggs and sugar until pale. Sift flour into the bowl. Add lemon juice and rind. Add milk and egg yolks. Whisk egg whites until they form stiff peaks. Fold gently into the egg yolk mixture. Pour into a buttered oven-proof dish. Bake in a pre-heated 180 C oven for 25-30 minutes until golden on top. The pudding has a warm citrus sauce underneath.

Perfect Upside Down Cake

Serves: 6

Ingredients

2/3 cup sugar

1/2 cup water

1 cup fresh fruit (plums, raspberries, strawberries)

130g unsalted butter

1/2 cup caster sugar (fine granulated)

3/4 cup flour

1 tsp sodium-free baking powder

2 tbsp ground almonds

1 tbsp Cointreau liqueur or1 tsp vanilla extract

Method

Place sugar and water in a pan and stir over low heat until sugar dissolves. Increase heat and boil syrup until it turns golden. Pour into a greased cake tin 20 cm, coating the bottom of the tin.

Place fruit on top of the caramel.

Cream butter and sugar together. Add eggs. Beat well. Sift flour and baking powder. Fold into the egg mixture. Add almonds, liqueur or vanilla.
Spoon over the fruit. Bake in a preheated oven at 190 C for 40-45 minutes until golden. Cool a little.
Tip the cake out onto a serving plate. Serve warm.

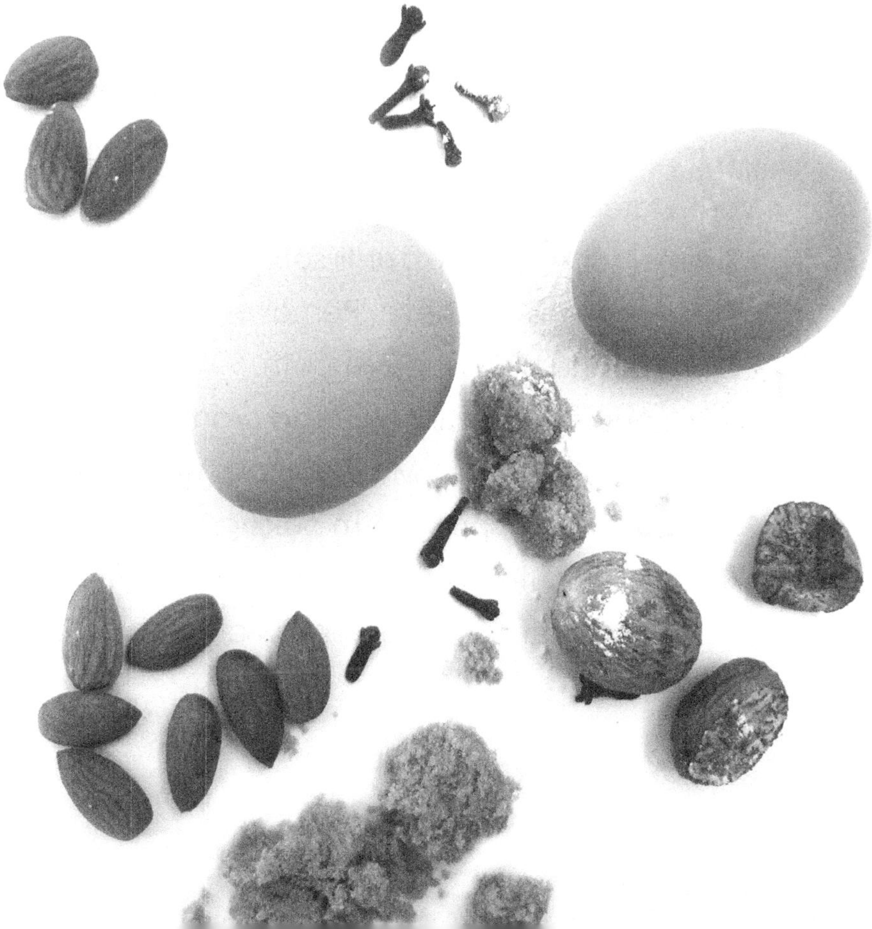

Sophia's Orange And Almond Pudding Cake

Ingredients

4 oranges, whole, skin on

6 eggs

3/4 cup granulated sugar

1 1/4 cups ground almonds

1 tsp sodium-free baking powder

Method

Wash oranges and place in a saucepan. Cover with water. Bring to the boil on medium heat. Tip out water. Replace with fresh water. Bring to boil. Simmer for 45 minutes, until soft.

Drain oranges in a sieve. Remove pips. Place in a blender and blend until smooth. Set aside. Beat eggs and sugar until pale. Add oranges, almonds and baking powder. Mix well. Pour into a lightly greased 18 cm spring-form baking tin. Bake at 180 C for 45 minutes to 1 hour. Test with a skewer. Cool cake in the tin. Remove from tin and serve.

Greek Island Shortbread

Ingredients

250g unsalted butter

50g sifted icing sugar (confectionery sugar)

300g sifted flour

100g, almonds, roasted and chopped

30 ml brandy, rum or whatever

1 tsp sodium-free baking powder

2 egg yolks

50g almond meal

Method

Beat butter and sugar until pale and fluffy. Beat in yolks and brandy. Stir in almonds and the rest of the dry ingredients. Mix with a fork until crumbly. Knead into a smooth dough. Break into walnut sized pieces. Roll and shape into crescents. Place on a greased baking sheet. Bake in a 160 C oven for 20 minutes or until lightly golden. Cool for 10 minutes. Dredge with a little icing sugar. Better on the second day if you can wait!

Warm Fruit Crumble

Serves: 6-8

Ingredients

1/3 cup plain (all purpose) flour

1 cup organic rolled oats

2/3 cup soft brown sugar

1 tsp mixed spice

1 tsp cinnamon

1 tbsp ground hazelnuts

1/2 cup walnuts or almonds, chopped

100g unsalted butter, softened

Fruit: 6 (granny smith) sweet green apples, peeled and thinly sliced mixed with 1/3 cup sugar and the pulp of 6 passionfruit.

You can also use combinations of fruit in this crumble. Just replace apples in the recipe with any of the following fillings: 2 cups stewed or pureed fruit in season. Rhubarb, plums, apricots, peaches or fresh berries.

Method

Preheat oven to 180 C. Place fruit in a buttered dish with 1/2 cup of the juice. Place remaining ingredients in a bowl. Using your fingers, 'crumble' the mixture until it resembles soft breadcrumbs. Place on top of fruit. Bake 40 minutes until crumbs are golden. Serve hot with Eve's vanilla custard.

Eve's Vanilla Custard

800 ml milk
2 tbsp plain flour
1 tsp cornflour
1/3 cup sugar
1 egg
1 tbsp unsalted butter
1 tsp unsalted butter (extra)
1 vanilla bean pod, cut in half length-ways

Method

Heat milk and vanilla bean slowly in a double boiler pan on low heat. Mix flour, sugar, cornflour, egg and butter in a bowl to make a thick paste. Add 3 tablespoons of the warm milk and whisk in. Add 3 more tablespoons to the paste. Whisk again. Do this again until you have a thin paste. Remove

vanilla pod from pan and scrape seeds with a knife. Discard pod and place seeds back into the milk. Add the thin paste to heated milk.
Stir until the custard starts to thicken. If becoming too thick, remove the pan from the heat. Keep stirring to avoid lumps. If you get a few lumps, whisk to remove them. Once thickness is achieved, add the teaspoon of butter and stir in. Serve immediately or cover in the fridge with plastic wrap. You can set this as a pudding; use in flans or in a ramekin as you would a crème caramel.

Health Benefits Of Vanilla:
Alleviates anxiety. Aphrodisiac properties. High levels of antioxidants help reduce free radicals in the body.

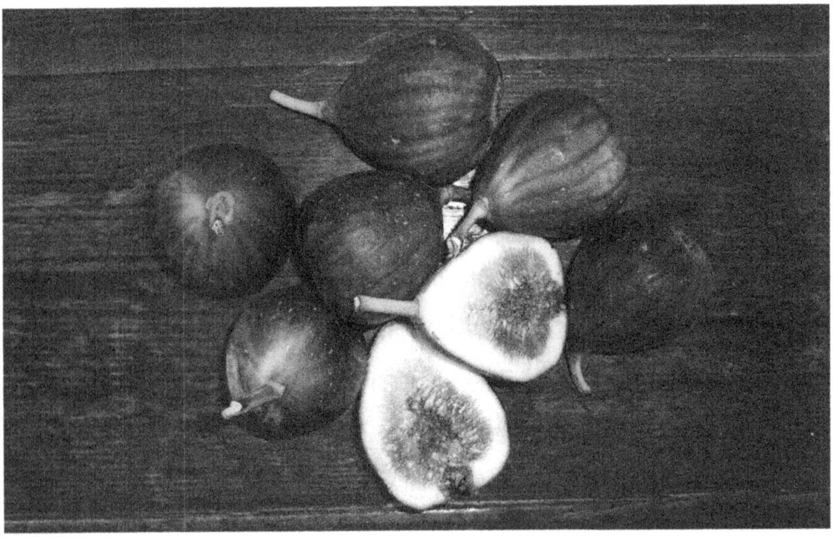

Sticky Date Pudding

Serves: 6-8

Ingredients

200g dates, pitted, chopped

1 cup boiling water

1 cup water

1 tsp low sodium bicarbonate of soda

100g unsalted butter

2/3 cup sugar (150g) caster sugar

2 large eggs, beaten

1 1/2 cup plain (organic) flour, sifted

1 1/2 tsp sodium-free baking powder

1/2 tsp vanilla essence

Cardamom Sauce:

100g brown sugar

1/2 cup cream

2 tbsp unsalted butter

4 cardamom pods, crushed

1 vanilla bean, split in half length-ways

Method To Make Sauce

Place ingredients for sauce in a saucepan. Bring to boil on medium heat. Reduce heat. Simmer for 5 minutes, stirring constantly.

Method

Heat oven to 180 C. Place dates in a bowl. Add bicarbonate of soda. Pour boiling water over. Let stand. Cream butter and sugar until pale. Beat in eggs. Fold in flour. Stir in dates and vanilla. Pour into a buttered cake tin, 18 cm square.

Bake for 30-40 minutes until firm. Cut pudding into serving squares. Remove vanilla bean and cardamom pods from sauce. Pour sauce over the pudding and serve.

Health Benefits Of Dates:

High in fiber. Low in fat. Supports healthy heart function.

Orange Poppy Seed Muffins

Makes 12

Ingredients

2 1/2 cups (310g) flour

2 tsp sodium-free baking powder

1/3 cup poppy seeds

1/3 cup caster sugar

125g (4oz) unsalted butter

2/3 cup orange (or lime) marmalade

1 cup (250ml) milk

2 eggs

Method

Heat oven to 200 C. Grease 12 muffin tins with unsalted butter. Sift flour with baking powder. Stir in poppy seeds and sugar. Make a well in the flour. Set aside. Place butter and marmalade in a saucepan. Cook over low heat until butter melts. Remove from heat. Cool slightly. Whisk eggs and milk together. Pour into the well in the flour. Add butter marmalade mixture. Carefully fold together until just moistened. Take care not to over mix or the muffins will go tough. The batter should be lumpy. Spoon into muffin tin. Bake 20-30 minutes until risen and golden. Cool in tin a few minutes. Loosen with a knife and cool on a wire rack.

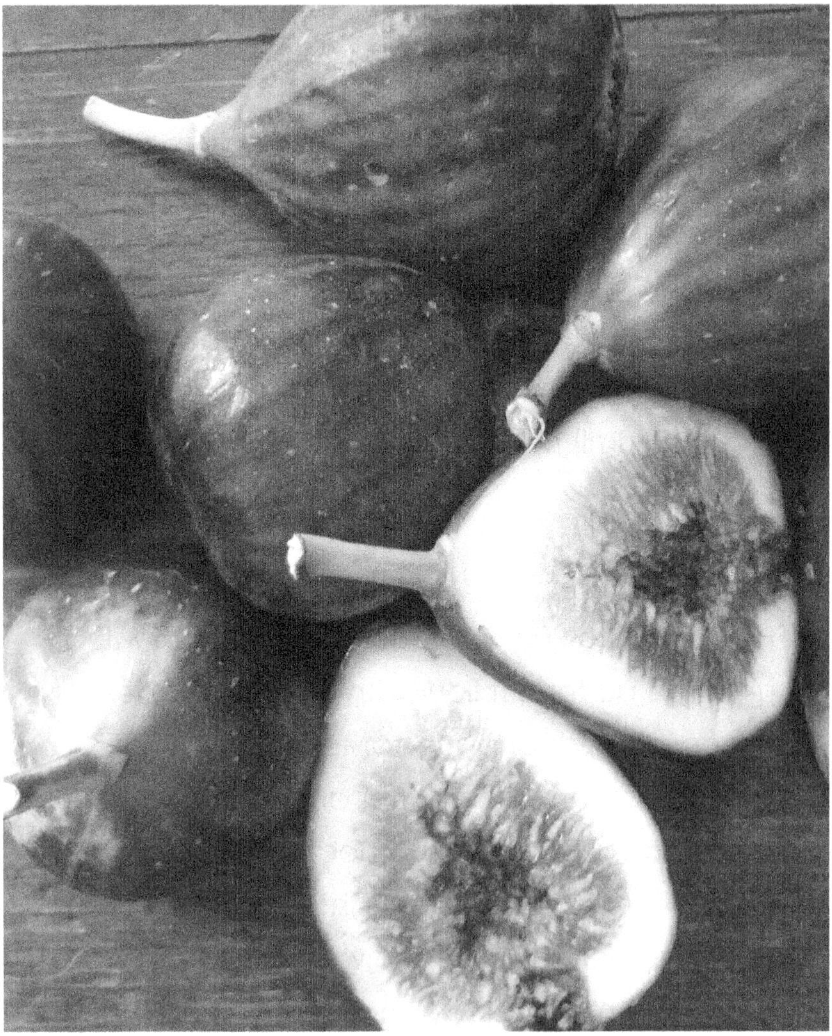

Orange And Date Muffins

Makes: 12

Ingredients

2 whole oranges

1 cup chopped dates

1 cup orange juice

250g unsalted butter, melted

2 eggs

3 cups plain flour

1 cup sugar

2 tsp sodium-free baking powder

Method

Heat oven to 200 C. Grease 12 muffin tins. Sift flour with baking powder. Stir in sugar. Set aside. Melt butter. Leave to cool slightly. Whisk eggs and orange juice together. Pour into flour. Add oranges and dates. Mix until just moistened. Spoon into muffin tin. Bake 20-30 minutes until golden brown.

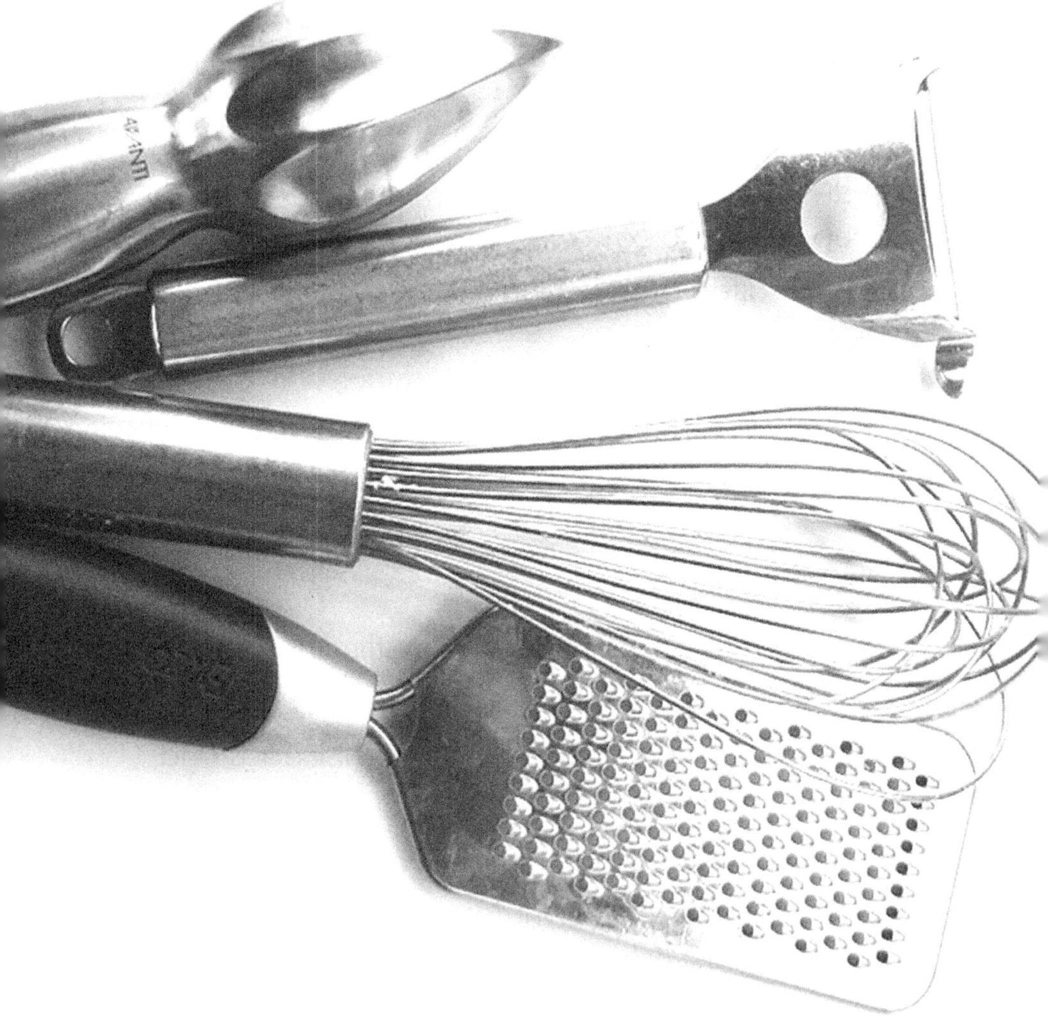

Lemon Muffins

Makes: 12

Ingredients

1 cup plain flour

1/2 cup sugar

1 heaped tsp sodium-free baking powder

1/4 cup unsalted butter, melted

2 eggs

1/2 cup freshly squeezed lemon juice

grated zest 1 lemon

Method

Heat oven to 190 C. Sift flour, baking powder, and sugar together. Remove melted butter from heat and allow to cool. Stir eggs, lemon juice and lemon zest into melted butter. Stir only enough to moisten the dry ingredients. Spoon into greased muffin tins. Bake for 15 minutes.

Bran Muffins

Makes: 12

Ingredients

1 cup flour

1/2 cup bran

1/2 cup wheat germ

1/2 cup raw sugar

125g melted butter

1 large egg

1/2 tsp mixed spice

1 tsp cinnamon

1 tsp sodium-free baking powder

1 cup raisins or sultanas

1 small cup apple pulp or mashed banana

Method

Place dry ingredients into a bowl Add beaten egg, fruit pulp and melted butter. Mix until just moist. Bake 190 C for 20-25 minutes, until muffins spring back when pressed,

Apricot And Walnut Muffins

Makes: 12

Ingredients

2 cups plain flour

1 tsp sodium-free baking powder

1 cup brown sugar

1 tsp cinnamon

1/2 cup chopped dried apricots

1/4 cup water or orange juice

100g unsalted butter

2 large eggs

1 cup yogurt

1 large orange, rind grated

juice of orange

1/2 cup chopped walnuts

Method

Place dry ingredients into a bowl. Mix well. Cook apricots with water or juice until liquid is absorbed. Remove from heat. Add butter. Mix in eggs, yogurt and orange rind. Add juice of orange plus enough water to equal a cup of liquid. Add walnuts. Fold together until just mixed. Take care not to over mix. Spoon mixture into greased muffin tins. Bake 190 C for 12-15 minutes or until muffins spring back when pressed and the tops are golden brown.

Health Benefits Of Apricots:
Contains vitamin C, copper, fiber and potassium.

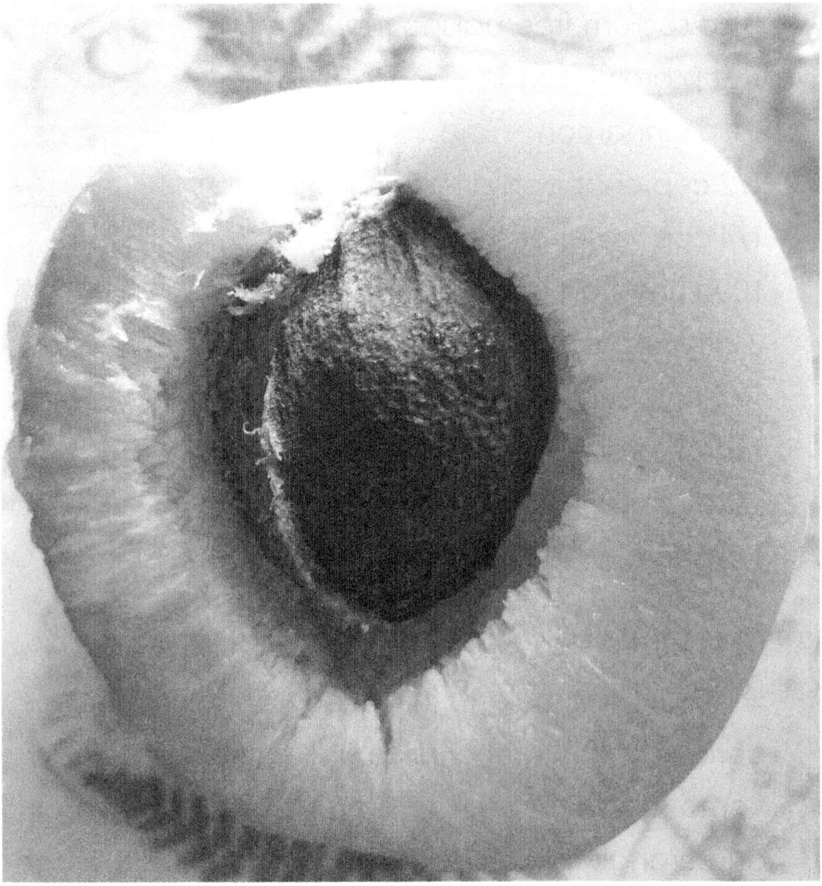

Blueberry Muffins

Makes: 12

Ingredients

1/2 cup (100g) brown sugar

60g unsalted butter, melted

1 egg

1 tsp vanilla essence

1/2 cup (125 ml) buttermilk

1 cup (125g) blueberries

1 1/2 cups (225g) plain organic flour

1 tsp sodium-free baking powder

1 1/2 tsp cinnamon

Method

Heat oven to 220 C. Grease 12 muffin tins.

Beat sugar, butter, egg, vanilla and buttermilk together. Sift flour, spices and baking powder together. Add egg mixture and fold lightly until just moistened. Fold in blueberries carefully. Take care not to over mix. Spoon into prepared baking tin. Bake for 20 minutes or until firm to touch.

Earl Grey Tea Cake

Ingredients

275g mixed dried fruit

60g soft dark brown sugar

300 ml fresh brewed decaffeinated black tea

275g organic plain flour

2 large eggs

2 1/2 tsp sodium-free baking powder

1 1/2 tsp cinnamon

1/2 tsp ground ginger

zest of 1/2 orange, grated

1/4 tsp grated nutmeg

Method

Heat oven to 170 C. Grease a loaf tin. Put fruit and tin a saucepan. Bring to boil. Simmer 1 minutes. Add sugar. Stir. Leave to cool. Add zest and eggs. Combine flour, spices and baking powder in a bowl. Add to fruit mixture. Pour into the baking tin. Bake 50-55 minutes. Cool in tin. Serve thickly sliced with plenty unsalted butter and hot Earl Grey Tea.

Apple Slice

Makes: 15 squares

Ingredients

8 eating apples (green skin) peeled, diced

1/2 cup (60g) cornflour

1 cup (150g) plain flour

1 tsp sodium-free baking powder

2 tbsp sugar

2 tbsp unsalted butter

1/2 cup water

1 egg yolk

cornflour for dusting

melted unsalted butter

sugar and cinnamon for topping

Method

Heat oven to 180 C. Line a baking tray with baking paper (18cm x 28cm). Place apples in a saucepan with a little water. Cook on low heat until soft. Drain. Cool. Sift flour and baking powder with cornflour. Add sugar. Rub in butter. Mix to a stiff dough with water and egg yolk to moisten.

Divide dough into two pieces. Roll out one piece and place in bottom of prepared tin. Sprinkle with a little cornflour to stop the base going soggy. Spread apple over base. Sprinkle top of apples with a little more cornflour. Roll our top and place over apples. Bake for 20 minutes. Remove from oven. Brush top with melted butter. Sprinkle with cinnamon and sugar. Cut into squares when cool.

Health Benefits Of Apples:
Soluble fiber helps insulin levels by releasing sugar slowly into the bloodstream. Cleanses and detoxifies the body and helps eliminate heavy metals like mercury and lead. Lowers cholesterol levels. Contains no fat or sodium. Excellent source of potassium, vitamin C, A and flavonoids.

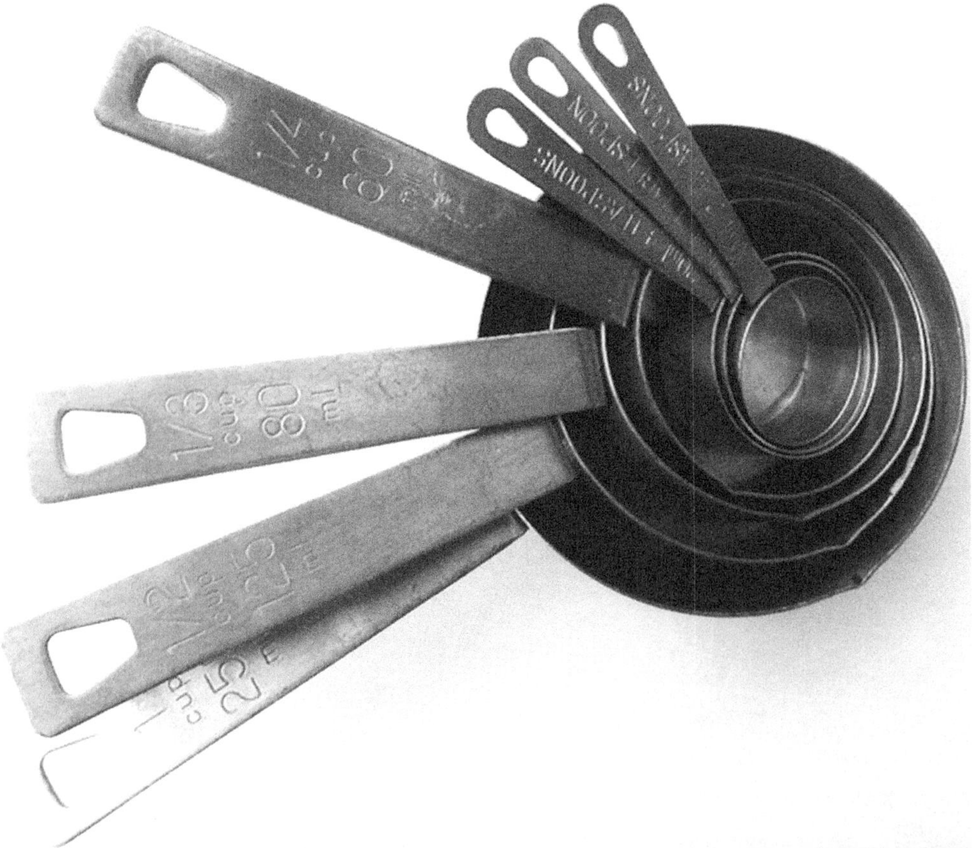

MEASUREMENTS

Oven Temperatures

Degree F		Degree C
200	=	100
225	=	110
250	=	120
275	=	140
300	=	150
325	=	160
350	=	180
375	=	190
400	=	200
425	=	220
450	=	230
475	=	240

Liquid Measures

1 tsp	=	5 mls
1 tbsb	=	20 mls
4 cups	=	1 liter
1/2 cup	=	125 mls

Solid measures

32 oz	=	1 kilogram
16 oz	=	500 grams
8oz	=	250 grams
7oz	=	220 grams
6 oz	=	185 grams
5 oz	=	155 grams
4 oz	=	125 grams
3 oz	=	90 grams
2 oz	=	60 grams
1 oz	=	30 grams

Glossary

Al Dente: Cooked until tender but firm to the bite. A term used to describe perfectly cooked pasta.

Baking Soda: Bicarbonate of soda, raising agent. Substitute regular baking soda for sodium-free baking soda. Low sodium content baking soda is available in supermarkets, specialty food stores and health food stores.

Baking Powder: Most commercial baking powders contain sodium aluminum sulphate, although brands such as Haine Featherweight Baking Powder *contain 0 mg per 1/4 teaspoon*.

You can make a baking powder substitute at home by mixing 1/2 teaspoon cream of tartar with 1/4 teaspoon of low sodium baking soda. Use to replace 1 teaspoon of baking powder in recipes. There is a site selling sodium-free and low sodium products online at healthyheartmarket.com.

Beetroot: Beets.

Balsamic Vinegar: A superior vinegar using a centuries old Italian technique. Aromatic, spicy and sweet sour taste.

Borlotti Beans: Small, speckled beans that are pale pinkish in color.

Bulgur Wheat: Dried cracked wheat.

Buttermilk: Makes baking lighter. You can make you own version simply by mixing 1 cup of milk and 1 tbsp of lemon juice.

Cake Tin: Cake/baking pan.

Chickpeas: Garbanzo beans.

Citrus Zest: The finely grated rind of citrus fruit.

1 lime = 1 tsp (teaspoon) of grated zest; 1 lemon = 2 tsp zest; l orange = 1 tbsp (tablespoon) zest; the juice of 1 lime = about 2 tbsp and the juice of 1 lemon = 4 tbsp or 1/4 cup.

Cos Lettuce: Romaine lettuce.

Coriander: Cilantro.

Cornflour: Cornstarch.

Creme Fraiche: Similar in flavor to sour cream. Used in both sweet and savory dishes.

Essence: Extract.

Eggplant: Aubergine.

Flour: Plain = standard flour.

Frying Pan: Skillet/frypan.

Ginger: 2 cm ginger root = 1 tsp finely grated ginger or 1 tbsp roughly grated.

Green Prawns: Raw prawns. Keep a bag in the freezer for quick meals.

Grill: Broil. To cook under the top oven element, or on the barbecue grill.

Hard-boiled Egg: Hard-cooked egg.

Icing Sugar: Confectioners sugar.

Kaffir Lime Leaves: Dark green glossy leaves add a citrus flavor. Shred and add to Asian style dishes.

King Prawns: Jumbo shrimp/scampi.

Lemongrass: A thick stalk with fragrant flavor. Easily found in most supermarkets. Be sure to peel away the tough outer layers of the stalk and use the tender parts.

Mascarpone: A fresh Italian cream cheese that can be used in both sweet and savory dishes. Follow the recipe in the book to save money and make your own salt free version at home.

Minced Meat: Ground meat

Mozzarella: Italian style cheese. See the recipe in this book and make your own at home.

Oven Temperatures: Oven temperatures vary depending if your oven is fan baked or not. Use cooking times as a guide. Check oven-baked dishes during cooking when trying a recipe for the first time. Always preheat your oven to start.

Passata: A brand name for tomatoes that have been skinned, deseeded and pulped. Usually sold in tall glass jars. It is the same type of puree you get if you mash canned tomatoes with a fork.
Pine Nuts: Seeds of the stone pine. Small, nutty and creamy tasting. Buy in small quantities and keep in the fridge to prevent them going rancid.
Polenta: Corn maize from Italy. Rich and golden in color. Milder than cornmeal with a smooth texture. Red kidney beans can be used instead. Soak all dried beans overnight before cooking.
Pomegranate Molasses: Specialty ingredient from delicatessens and supermarkets.
Ricotta Cheese: Soft curd, low fat cheese. Use in savory and sweet dishes. Make your own ricotta by using the recipe in this book.
Rocket: Arugula, rocquette, rucola, rugula.
Roma Or Plum Tomatoes: Egg-shaped tomatoes with plenty of juicy flesh and a few seeds. Ideal for making sauces. My preference is for Italian style Roma tomatoes as they are less acidic. Add a pinch of sugar where tomatoes are acid. Always chose robust, flavorsome, ripe and red. A truss of organic tomatoes, fully ripened gives more obvious flavor to food than pale force ripened ones.

Seed: Pip.

Shallots: Small sized onions with a sweeter taste than regular onions. Delicious whole or roasted. can be chopped and added to sauces and salsas.

Simmer: To cook just under poiling point- small bubbles may erupt in one place.

Smokey Paprika: A spice made from ground capsicums(bell peppers). Adds a smoky flavor and to BBQ grilled or roasted meat, chicken and vegetables. The Spanish paprika is the smoked variety called *Pimenton* and is available in sweet *(dulce)*, moderate or sweet and sour *(agridulce)* and spicy *(picante)*.

Spring Onions: Green onions or scallions.

Steam: To cook food in a rising steam.

Stock: Enriched 'cooking water' produced from simmering stock ingredients. Using homemade no salt stock from fresh ingredients makes all the difference to your cooking.

Sweet Peppers: Capsicum/bell peppers.

Thai Basil: A stronger, peppery flavor compared to Italian basil. Used in Asian style dishes.

Tomato Products: Canned Italian tomatoes are a superior product, rich, sweet and full of flavor. Buy reduced sodium or no salt cans.

Turmeric: An aromatic spice from the same family as the ginger root plant, so you can use it in the same way. Adds color and warm peppery flavor.

Vanilla: Use natural vanilla extract where possible. Use vanilla bean pods when heating milk. Scrape out the seeds and use with flavored milk for custards and desserts. Keep a pod in a jar of sugar to make vanilla sugar for baking and desserts.

Vermicelli Noodles: Thin noodles made from rice. Hydrate in water before you use. Add to salads and stir fries.

Meniere Man Books

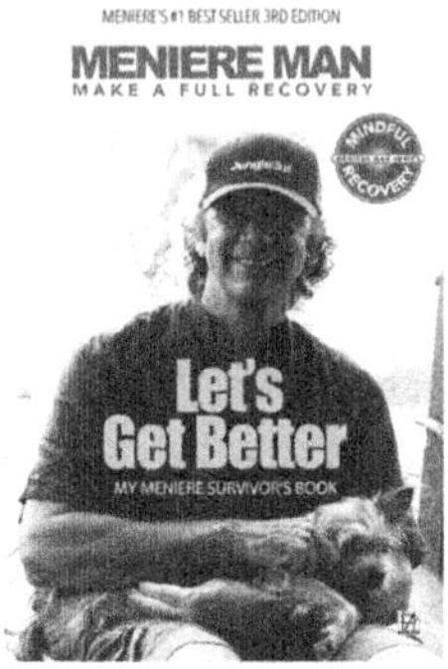

Let's Get Better

A Memoir of Meniere's Disease

From Meniere Sufferer to Meniere Survivor.

A truly remarkable and successful recovery story.

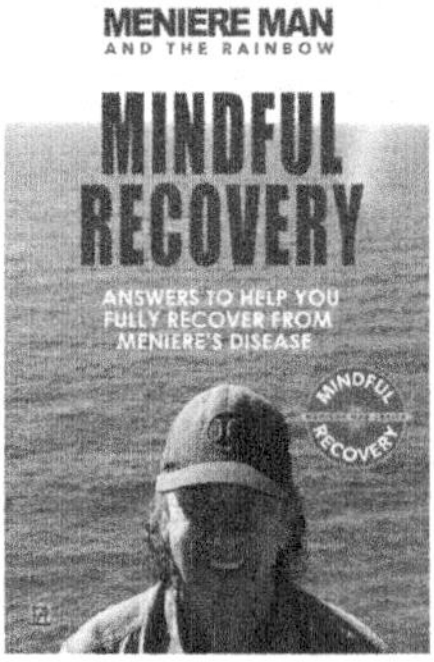

Meniere Man And The Rainbow

Answers to Help You Fully Recover From Meniere's

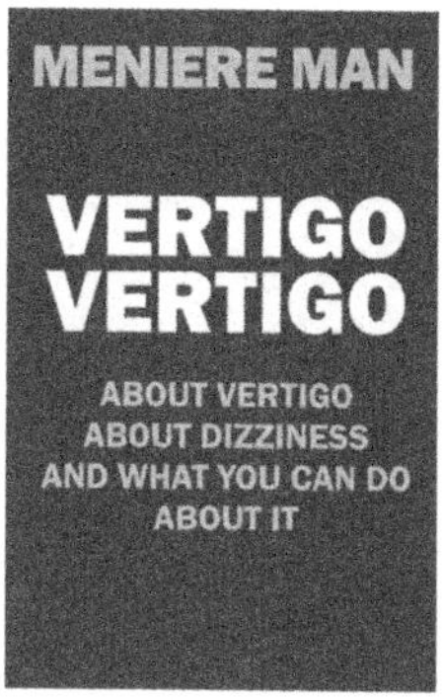

Vertigo Vertigo

About Vertigo About Dizziness and What You Can Do About it.

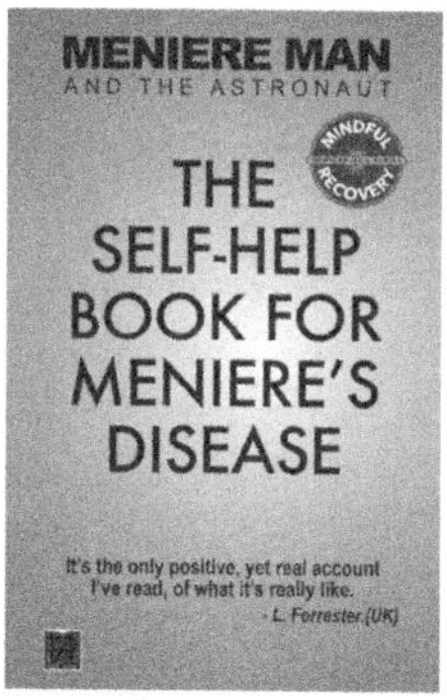

Meniere Man And The Astronaut
The Self Help Book for Meniere's Disease

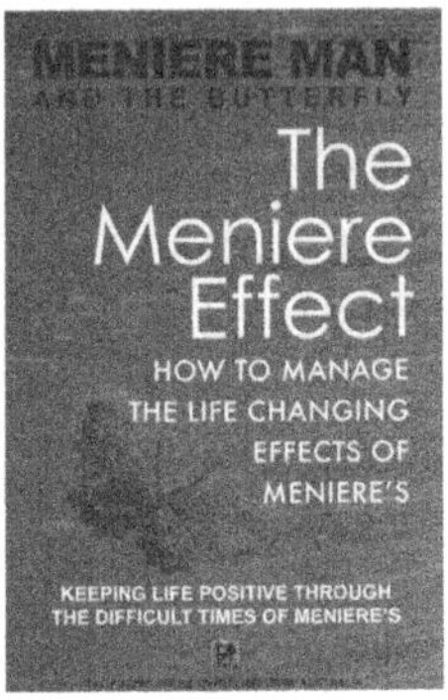

Meniere Man And The Butterfly.
The Meniere Effect

How to Manage the Life Changing Effects of Meniere's

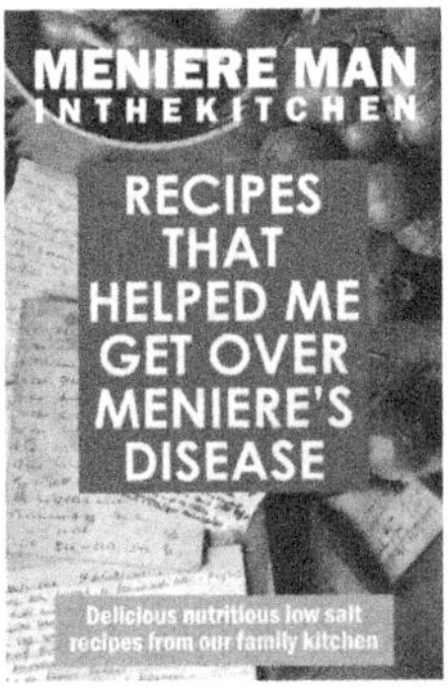

Recipes That Helped Me Get Over Meniere's

Delicious nutritious low salt recipes from our family kitchen. Book 1

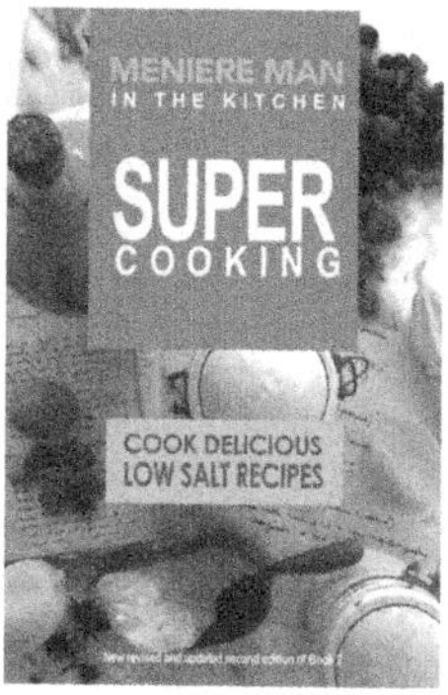

**Meniere Man Super Cooking.
Cook delicious Low Salt Recipes**

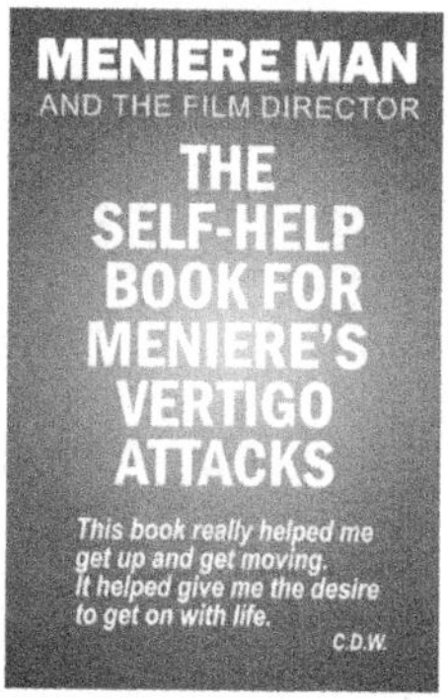

The Self Help Book for Meniere's Vertigo Attacks.

How to cope: Before, During, and After vertigo attacks.
Real, practical, helpful advice.

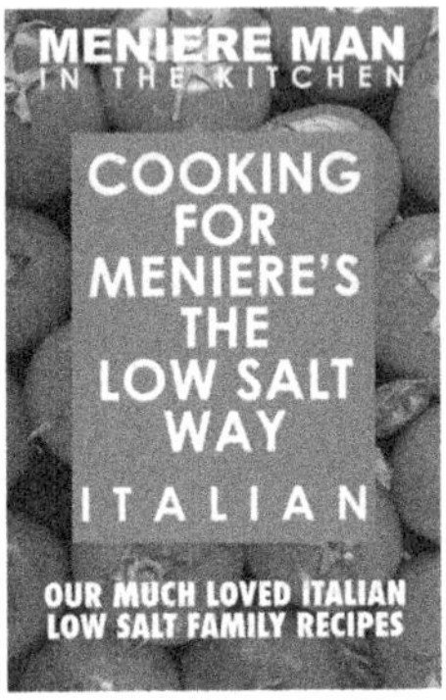

Meniere Man In The Kitchen.
Cooking For Meniere's The Low Salt Way.
Italian.

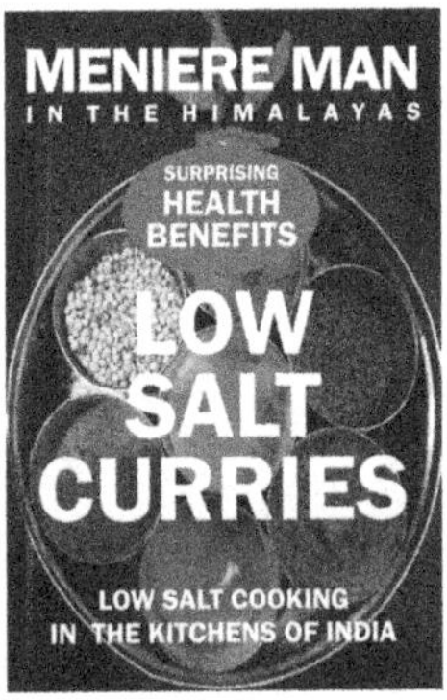

Meniere Man In The Himalayas.
Low Salt Curries

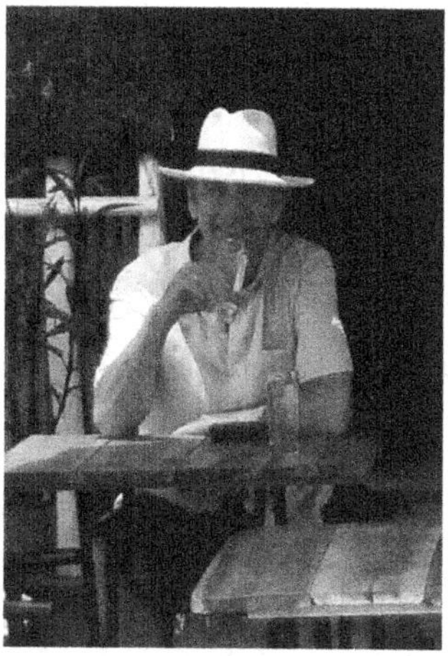

About The Author

At the height of his business career, the author was diagnosed with Meniere's disease, but the full impact of having Meniere's disease was to come later. He was to lose not only his health, but his career. He began to lose all hope that he would fully recover a sense of well-being. But it was his personal spirit and desire to get 'back to normal' that made him not give up to a life of Meniere's symptoms of severe vertigo, dizziness and nausea.

He decided that you can't put a limit on anything in life. Rather than letting Meniere's disease get in the way of recovery, he focused on what to do about overcoming Meniere's disease.

These days life is different for the Author. He is a fit active man who has no symptoms of Meniere's disease except for hearing loss and tinnitus in one ear. Following his own advice he continues to avoid salt, stress, takes vitamins, exercises regularly and maintains a positive, mindful attitude. He does not take any medication.

All the physical activities he enjoys these days require a high degree of balance and equilibrium: snowboarding, surfing, hiking, windsurfing, weightlifting, and riding a motorbike.

Meniere Man believes that if you want to experience a marked improvement in health you can't wait until you feel well to start. You must begin to improve your health now, even though you don't feel like it.

The Author is a writer, painter, designer and artist. He is married to a poet. They have two adult children. He spends most days writing or painting. He enjoys the sea, cooking, travel, photography, nature and the great company of family, friends and his beloved dog, Bella.

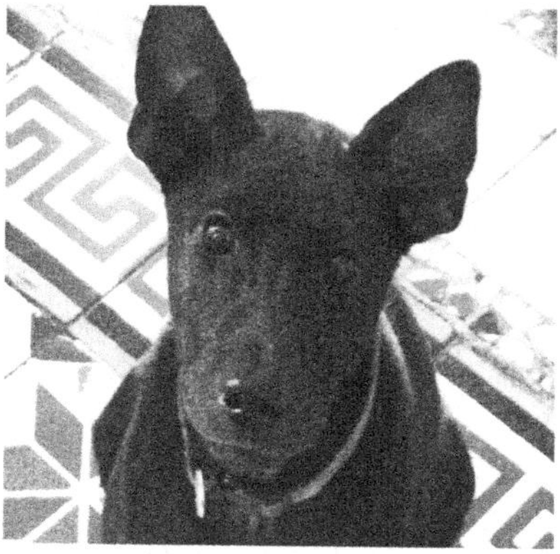

Additional Information

If you enjoyed this Meniere Man book and you think it could be helpful to others, please leave a review for the book. Thank you.

Meniere Support Networks

Meniere's Society (UNITED KINGDOM)
www. menieres.org.uk
Meniere's Society Australia (AUSTRALIA)
info@menieres.org.au
The Meniere's Resource & Information Centre (AUSTRALIA)
www.menieres.org.au
Healthy Hearing & Balance Care (AUSTRALIA)
www.healthyhearing.com.au
Vestibular Disorders association (AUSTRALIA)
www.vestibular .org
The Dizziness and Balance Disorders Centre (AUSTRALIA)
www.dizzinessbalancedisorders.com
Meniere's Research Fund Inc (AUSTRALIA)
www.menieresresearch.org.au
Australian Psychological Society APS (AUSTRALIA)
www.psychology.org.au
Meniere's Disease Information Center (USA)
www.menieresinfo.com
Vestibular Disorders Association (USA)
www.vestibular.org
BC Balance and Dizziness Disorders Society (CANADA)
www.balanceand dizziness.org
Hearwell (NEW ZEALAND)
www.hearwell.co.nz
WebMD.
www.webmd.com
National Institute for Health
www.medlineplus.gov
Mindful Living Program
www.mindfullivingprograms.com
Center for Mindfulness
www. umassmed.edu.com

Made in the USA
Monee, IL
04 November 2026

67374653R00134